WHAT ARE YU WAITING FOR?

Still to this day I remember Mr. Hauswirth taking me up to the gym at school, looking at me, and telling me "you have to come in with a purpose; you need to make every workout count." I have lived with that motto ever since. When I was struggling with every rep and it was burning, it hurt, and I couldn't push anymore, he'd tell me, "push it Mohler, make it count." Now when I'm struggling, I'm on my last wind, and I can't push anymore, I hear "push it Mohler make it count." That saying has gotten me past more lock-out points and last reps than I care to count. So when you've decided enough is enough and you're ready to get serious..."make it count."

—A1C Paul Mohler USAF

I've known Jeff for two years, and he is passionate about helping young people. This book is a great entry level guide geared to give basic concepts on weight training. Jeff makes these concepts easy to understand and gives you practical information you can utilize right away. This book will help start you in the right direction to live a healthier life.

—Heather Reinke,
Assistant Athletic Director,
Head Women's Ice Hockey Coach,
Finlandia University

WHAT ARE YOU WAITING FOR?

JEFF HAUSWIRTH

WHAT ARE YOU WAITING FOR?

A BEGINNER'S GUIDE TO WEIGHT TRAINING

TATE PUBLISHING
AND ENTERPRISES, LLC

What are you Waiting For?
Copyright © 2012 by Jeff Hauswirth. All rights reserved.

No part of this publication may be reproduced, stored in a retrieval system or transmitted in any way by any means, electronic, mechanical, photocopy, recording or otherwise without the prior permission of the author except as provided by USA copyright law.

This book is designed to provide accurate and authoritative information with regard to the subject matter covered. This information is given with the understanding that neither the author nor Tate Publishing, LLC is engaged in rendering legal, professional advice. Since the details of your situation are fact dependent, you should additionally seek the services of a competent professional.

The opinions expressed by the author are not necessarily those of Tate Publishing, LLC.

Published by Tate Publishing & Enterprises, LLC
127 E. Trade Center Terrace | Mustang, Oklahoma 73064 USA
1.888.361.9473 | www.tatepublishing.com

Tate Publishing is committed to excellence in the publishing industry. The company reflects the philosophy established by the founders, based on Psalm 68:11,
"The Lord gave the word and great was the company of those who published it."

Book design copyright © 2012 by Tate Publishing, LLC. All rights reserved.
Cover design by Shawn Collins
Interior design by Chelsea Womble

Published in the United States of America

ISBN: 978-1-61862-945-6
1. Health & Fitness / Exercise
2. Health & Fitness / General
12.05.14

This book is dedicated to my mom, Janet Louise
Hauswirth, the toughest person I ever met.
June 20, 1943—August 24, 2008
Live, Love, be Happy.

ACKNOWLEDGMENTS

There are so many people who have helped make me who I am today and helped to bring me to this point. If you had asked me even a year ago if I were to ever write a book, I would have not thought it possible. I owe to my parents, Janet and Lee, the attitude to never quit, no matter what. Their love was always there. Thank you to my brothers, Bill (thanks for that first pep talk), Mike, and David, who have always been there. I will always be there for you guys. To my lovely wife, Erin, whose support has been nonstop. Erin is also my female example in the book. To my kids, Tyler, Kaitlin and Megan, who are the reason I push to stay young.

To Jim Luoma, who, as a coach, pushed me to be my best, always. To Ken Klein, whose knowledge of the weight room and the football field helped me grow as an educator, a coach, and a person. To Dr. Randy Jensen at Northern Michigan University, you don't know it, but you made learning Kinesiology and Physiology cool for me. Thank you also to Thomas

Schmidt (my male example in this book) for being a great person and student, as well as a great example of how to lift properly. Thank you also to LaVayeda McClellan and to Jordan Jaehnig for helping me make sure this all makes sense.

To my military family all over the world, wherever you are, I support what you do. To Abe and Richie, whose workouts in Iraq I will never forget… there's something about pumping iron when it's 140 degrees outside!

There are so many to thank that there could be a separate book written. I would like to thank the staff at Tate Publishing for giving me this opportunity to say what I have to say. Lastly, I would like to thank you, the reader of this book. It is my hope that what you are about to read fits your needs. Bless you all for giving me and this book an opportunity.

TABLE OF CONTENTS

FOREWORD **15**

A LITTLE ABOUT ME **16**

WHY GET STARTED? **19**

STARTING POINTS **22**

GOALS **28**

THE ART OF LIFTING **31**

THE WORKOUT **33**
   THE GREAT 8 WORKOUT **33**
     Muscle Groups and Choices 34
       Group One 34
       Group Two 36

HOW IT WORKS **38**

STARTING EACH WORKOUT **41**

LET'S DO THIS! 43

GROUP ONE STRETCHES 43
Neck Stretch 45
Sky Scraper 46
Wall Stretch...47
Trunk Twist..48
Overhead Bent Arm 49
Static Hugger 50
Straight Arm Clasp 51
Reverse Straight Arm Clasp 52

CHEST... 53
Bench Press 53
Incline Bench Press..55
Dumbbell Flies 56
Dumbbell Press..58
Pec Deck Fly Machine 60
Three Stage Pushups 62

TRICEPS 65
Dips 65
Throw Backs 67
Triceps Push Downs...68
Close Grip Bench Press 69
Nose Breakers 70
Overhead Triceps 71

SHOULDERS 73
Military Press...73
Lateral Raises 75
Bent Over Flies..76
Front Raises...78

Barbell Raises 80
Wide Grip Upright Rows 81
Shrugs 82

BICEPS 84
Preacher Curls 84
One-Arm Standing Full Supination Curls 86
Hammer Curls 88
21s 90
Isolation Curls 93
Standing Wall Curls 94
Ten-Second Curls 95

GROUP TWO STRETCHES 97
Hamstring Stretch 97
Groin Stretch 99
Standing Quad Stretch 100
Side Stretch 101
Cobra Stretch 102
Cat Stretch 103

LATS 104
Lawn Mowers 104
Lat Pull Downs 106
Straight Arm Pull Downs 108
Bent Over Rows 110
Reverse Grip Bent Over Rows 112
Seated Rows 113

QUADS 114
Leg Extension 114
Wall Sits 116
Dumbbell Squat 118

Hamstring ... 120
- Leg Curls ... 120
- Straight Leg Dead Lift ... 121
- Good Mornings ... 123
- Flutter Kicks ... 124

Leg Combo ... 126
- Squats ... 126
- Plyometric Jumps ... 128
- Lunges ... 130
- Side Lunges ... 132

Abdominals ... 134
- Russian Twists ... 135
- Feet Up Crunch ... 137
- Leg Lifts ... 139
- Bicycle Twist Crunch ... 140
- Heel Lifts ... 142
- Side Crunch ... 143
- Leg Climb ... 144

Variation ... 146

And Finally... ... 151

Appendix ... 153
Group One Lifts ... 154
Group Two Lifts ... 156

FOREWORD

I remember Jeff and I being the only two guys in the gym at these huge military bases. We were so into our workouts that neither of us would say more than a sentence or two to each other. We would be ridiculed by our fellow shipmates for working out and running the day or night before a bi-annual physical fitness test.

My body is in relative shambles from years of doing it wrong. When I started working out little thought was given to fundamentals of kinesiology and body mechanics. As I write this foreword I am recovering from my third shoulder surgery. After playing high school sports, spending ten years in the navy, and now working as a firefighter paramedic, I find that I should have read a book like this twenty years ago, or at least listened to my body more intently.

—Shane Clifton
EMT/Paramedic, SPFD St. Paul, Minnesota
United States Navy, 1998-2007

A LITTLE ABOUT ME

I am going to be up front. I do not consider myself an "expert." I do not have a PhD or fancy, meaningful letters of any kind after my name (although I do have a Bachelors and I am a middle school teacher). I won't tell you that this program will be the greatest thing ever…in the whole world…since the beginning of mankind. I won't tell you that this will be easy or done quickly. Results will vary depending on your work ethic and motivation to change. There is no fast and simple way to change you physically. Any diet, exercise program, or piece of equipment that tells you otherwise isn't worth purchasing. No matter what you choose, you have to put the work in to get results.

Over the years, I have found (at least for me) through trial and error what works and what is a "baloney sandwich." I have also found that it is easier to stick to a program when there is a definite plan in place and a goal to accomplish, not only long term, but day to day. So, why sit and do this? Why write a book? Well, I have life experience. I have been there, wishing I had direction, and I know this works. I have tried many programs that will make this or that promise. I have also wasted a lot of money on this product or that product that "guarantees" results. Well, the bottom-line for results comes down to two things: *your* work ethic and *your* motivation to change.

That is what this program that I lay before you is. It will hopefully give you direction, help you to plan those daily and long term goals, and get you started on a path to weight training. Where you go from here is only limited by your work ethic. I know that there are a *ton* more lifts than what is here, but to me getting started isn't about being fancy. If, as time goes on, you change up your routine and add some of the more complicated exercises, that's up to you. I am not saying they are good or bad. What I am saying by writing this is that you can do this. You can get started on a path to change the way you look and feel. You can become a healthier you for life.

I will never forget the first time that I went to a weight room. It was the summer before my freshman year of high school. I had big plans of walking in and lifting everything that weight room had, and then turning into a massive football star at my high school. To say the least, that's not exactly what happened. My first experience in the weight room lasted about three minutes. You see, I went with my oldest brother, who just happened to be a college football player, and we went to workout at his gym (the college weight room). I was working out with these *massive* people. Folks who obviously ate kids my size for a snack. I watched a couple guys on the bench press, and then it was my turn. I figured I would warm up with ninety-five pounds on the bench press and about burst a capillary in my brain trying to push it up. I immediately got up, figured everyone was laughing at me, and I walked out. I was content to sit in the locker room for the rest of my life and never be seen again.

Lucky for me, my brother followed me, and he began to teach me a very important lesson that day. We *all* have to start somewhere, and these "walking trees" didn't start out bench pressing compact cars. I was lucky to have that pep talk from him, although I am sure he doesn't remember it the same way.

So I am writing this from experience. From the experience of one who has been in and out of the weight room (mostly in) for over twenty-eight years. Not everything I have tried has worked, but I guarantee that this system will put you on a path of success *if you stay with it*! I am not going to guarantee results or that you will one day squat minivans, but I will tell you that if you stick with it, this program will give you a great base which you can build upon as you gain experience in the weight room.

I wrote this book as a beginner's guide, so it's pretty much for anyone who is around the age of thirteen and up who is looking to start a weight training regime for whatever reason. I have used this program to get many kids started on the right path. I have also used this same program with adults who have never set foot in a weight room, but know they need to get healthy. Stick with this. It will get you started.

WHY GET STARTED?

One question I hear a lot is *why*. "Why should I lift weights?" You can do the research, but physical fitness leads to many health benefits. The earlier you start a program, the better off you will be. Weight training, building and toning muscle, leads to things like lower cholesterol, decreased heart disease risks, a decreased risk in certain cancers, increased mood and concentration levels, increased stamina, increased metabolism, and an increase in the ability to handle stress, just to name a few.

If you happen to be younger, I know you are probably thinking "but all that stuff happens to old people!" Here is a news flash: *One day you will be older!* Believe it or not, parents weren't born old. Believe it or not, one day you will be heading towards middle age, and hopefully living a healthy lifestyle. Good habits for that healthy lifestyle are formed at a young age. So, if you are young, now is the time to develop those habits.

But, wait. What if you are older and are worried about those things listed above? Don't fret. It's not over for you. Starting to develop a healthier lifestyle can help you at any age. So if you are in that heading towards middle age group, there is hope. Nobody is too old to begin.

This leads to the question, "Well, okay, but how do I begin?" It really can be intimidating if you let it be. Part of losing that fear is to have a plan (as I mentioned before). Things will be a lot less complicated and intimidating if you know what you are getting into, whether it is lifting or any other facet of life. So I am (hopefully) creating a plan for you to get started, to keep you moving, and to change yourself in more than just a physical nature.

There are many myths that I hear from people who don't lift. One is that those who train with weights become muscle bound and lose flexibility. Not true. Flexibility, or lack thereof, comes from not stretching properly. Becoming muscle bound depends on how heavy a weight you lift. Science proves that for toning, you should use a light weight/high reps system and for strength, a heavier weight/low reps system. I will explain later how you can do either one with this beginning program.

Females who lift weights, for the most part, become harder; meaning their muscles will become much firmer before they become larger. Of course, there are those women who spend their whole lives lifting and power training, and (no pun intended) more power to them. I have nothing against that at all. The workout I am describing is a great starter plan for boys and girls, men and women. It is for anyone who wants to get into it.

That leads to another myth: the myth that lifting weights being for men only. Or ladies don't need to lift weights. Oh, really? Starting a resistance exercise program at an early age for a girl can help stave off osteoporosis by helping increase bone density. It is a proven fact that at a certain age (somewhere in the mid to late thirties), women's bodies stop using calcium as effectively and this can lead to bone thinning as they age. Lifting weights and resistance exercise can help increase bone density, giving them thicker bones to work with as they get older.

I have heard many more reasons as to why people shouldn't get into weight training. For the most part, they are myths and excuses from lazy people. In my most humble of opinions, somewhere around the start of puberty is the best time to develop these habits. Learn to love it early and it will stick with you forever.

STARTING POINTS

A very important factor here to keep in mind is to make sure you understand what you are doing before you jump in and do it. Think in your own life if there has ever been a time when you figured, "Yup, that's what I am going to do," and jumped in having no clue as to how things should or could go, wound up being frustrated, and just gave up. I am hoping I am not the only one in this category. So, along with having a plan and the right mindset, below are some thoughts that run through my mind that may help you as you get started.

Some things to keep in mind before beginning any program:

- Make sure you are physically able to exercise. This may seem a little goofy, because it's all over the news about how we all need to exercise more, but based on certain physical or congenital ailments, there are some people for whom it may be more harmful than helpful to exercise. Obviously, if you are involved in sports, you should pretty much be good for this. If you have had a physical and everything was okay, you should be good to go. Being mentally prepared is also key, so from day one plan for success!

- The object of this (or any) program is *consistency*. Starting and stopping a program, missing days, lame excuses (and most of them are), any of that type of stuff and you will see no gains or improvement. It takes a *minimum* of 3-5 weeks before you will notice any sort of improvement. This is where the frustration and quitting can creep in. Start now to discipline yourself to make this program happen *every day, no matter what*. Commit to weight training mentally, as well as physically. In the beginning, it will be your proper mind set as well as your self-discipline that leads to early gains. It is up to you, especially early on, to motivate yourself to get it done. Not to get too scientific, but somewhere within the first three weeks, your body goes through a neural growth phase. Basically, your muscle fibers begin to work more efficiently. Between that three to five week mark, you will start what is known as hypertrophy, where the fibers actually start to grow. I always laugh when I see those commercials on TV: "if you don't see improvement in six weeks, we will refund your money." Well, *duh*! No matter *what* program you do, you will see a change if you are consistent with it for at least six weeks!

- Exercise is only *part* of the equation. Proper rest, along with a proper diet, is imperative to this and any program. When we sleep is when our bodies send out the hormones to repair and build and grow our bodies. Lacking sleep is short-changing your workouts. Depending on your age, we all need somewhere between seven and nine hours of sleep a night. As well as sleep, we need to rest our muscles after a good workout so that they can properly recover. Don't think you will get a benefit from doing the same routine (working the same muscle groups) two days in a row. It will do more harm than good, so stick to the plan. Getting the proper fuel for your body is also as important. To spare you the details of what makes a proper diet, I *strongly* encourage you to check out www.myplate.gov. It is an excellent website. Surf around in there and see what you should be fueling up with and how much you should be fueling up with as well.

- Warming up and cooling down are also very important factors. They should be included as part of your workout and *never* skipped (I will describe some ideas later).

- The first two to three weeks will be the worst and will definitely test your faith to this new commitment. Anyone who says starting a program is easy is full of a lot more than boloney. If it is new to you, your body will react by arguing with you. You will be sore. You might feel a little run down. Your mind will try to convince you to stop. This is normal. As for the soreness, what is happening is known as delayed onset muscle soreness (DOMS). This is a natural reaction to increasing your workload. There is, however, a difference between a little sore and outright pain. If you have outright pain, it's probably best to be seen by a professional before continuing. Mostly, work through it, and you will be better off for it.

- Don't expect to move mountains your first time out. Don't be ashamed if there is someone around lifting more. It is not a competition. Actually, it sort of is, but the contestants are you versus you. *Your* best is what matters, especially when starting. What the person next to you is doing does not mean a whole lot to what you want to accomplish for yourself.

- It is also very important to have a positive mindset. As I stated earlier, had I gone with my original feeling when I entered my first weight room, you wouldn't be reading this. I was lucky enough to have someone boot me in the hind parts to get me going. Ever since then, I have had to do it myself. Especially when you begin, training with a partner can serve as a great motivator. You'll have someone to work out with and to help push you, to help challenge you both mentally and physically. Also, by training with a partner, you will always have a spotter on hand.

- Plan each workout *before* you get to the gym! Don't get there then think, "Well, I guess I should do…" Be efficient. I don't know of many people who would want to build a house or even a plastic model airplane without some sort of idea of how they want it to go. Your body is the same way. In your notebook, write down the lifts you want to do for that day (or copy and use the sheets at the end of this book and take them with you). You wouldn't build a house without a plan, why build your body without one?

- Lastly on this subject, *be honest with yourself!* Each day, when you work out, write down what you did, and how many you did…*exactly*! Keep a lifting logbook. Sometimes the easiest people to lie to are ourselves. I don't know why this is, but just because you write it down doesn't make it a fact. Don't develop the close enough attitude. It doesn't do you any good. Believe it or not, this happens. I would prefer to be honest with myself, regardless. In essence, no matter what you write, you will know, but keep it honest on paper and you will feel better, even if it's not where you wanted to be. It is usually the hardest to be honest with yourself, but the first step to achieving anything is facing reality. It is a *lot* easier to rely on what you wrote as far as how heavy a weight was and how many reps you had then it is to remember. It's also a good place to put your goals down, so you see them every time you work out. Sometimes, when you are in the middle of things, you can't see the growth, but having the ability to look at why you are exercising, and seeing over a period of time how you have improved helps to keep things clear and in perspective.

GOALS

Along with having a day-to-day plan for what to work on, another good idea for you is to set some goals for what you want to accomplish. Start lifting weights isn't really a goal. It's more of an idea or a proclamation. Think a little more long term and concrete. What do you want to accomplish by starting? What about when you reach that goal, then what? The day-to-day lifts in this book are great for planning a routine, but think a little farther out as for what you want. What are you aiming for down the road to keep you going from day to day? Setting goals will make it more personal for you. What do you want to accomplish by weight lifting? Do you want to gain size? Lift a certain amount? Do you want to lose some fat and gain some muscle? For some, a long-term goal could be a month from now. For others, it could be longer. The length can vary from person to person. When it comes to weight training, I try to set quarterly goals. Something like, "in three months, I want to be able to…" This will give you something to challenge yourself with on a daily basis. Don't just say them, either. Write them down. Keep them somewhere where you will see them on a regular basis (like your lifting log maybe).

Thinking along the lines of goal setting, when setting a long or short-term goal, keep two questions in mind: One, is this achievable? And two, how will I know when I have reached it (meaning is it measurable)? Part of the problem sometimes with goal setting is people don't really know when or if they have accomplished them. How will you really know when you get better or do more? Those types of words are hard to measure. So, pick something that you can do and something that you can measure. Sounds easy and in many respects it is, but some people have difficulty.

So here is an example: maybe for starters, a long-term goal could be something like "I want to still be training with weights on a regular basis in (fill in the blank) months." That's pretty easy. You would know if you are doing this. Whatever your long-term goal is, use the short-term goals as a stepping stone or the plan as to how to go about reaching that long-term goal. For this approach, your day-to-day lifts could serve as your short-term goals.

Something pretty unrealistic would be " I want to be bench pressing 500 pounds by next week." Obviously, that's an overstatement and overreach. Setting goals that are knowingly unattainable are just as bad as not setting any. Why, you ask? Well, for starters, it can lead to frustration and giving up. It can be the same for choosing something that is too easy. Finding the right match of challenging but achievable goals takes some time. Stick with it and you will find that balance. Don't sell yourself short. I can't stress enough the importance of writing this stuff down and referring to it on a regular basis.

Now, let's say you set a goal and it seems achievable and it is also measurable. You work towards it and for whatever reason it doesn't come to fruition. Now what? Obviously, don't quit! Sometimes we all fall short. So, maybe it's time to reevaluate. Did you maybe pick too lofty a goal? Did you maybe not work as hard as you thought to achieve it? Is it still worth striving for? Maybe you need more time. Either way, keep striving, keep setting the bar high, and keep working towards it.

THE ART OF LIFTING

Now, this part may seem a bit boring, but it is important that you fully understand the art of lifting before you jump into it. Proper technique is as important as it gets for safety, growth, and avoiding injury. You may want to read this a couple of times to make sure you understand, to help reduce injury.

With lifting, there are two movements of any muscle group: concentric movement (shortening or flexing a muscle) and eccentric movement (lengthening a muscle). This is important to things such as timing and when to breathe. It sounds funny, but yes, I have seen people who forget to breathe when lifting and not much good can come from that.

First, let's talk about timing. I like to use a four-count to two-count. During the eccentric phase of lifting you use a slower four-count pace. During the concentric movement, you explode into the lift and bring it to its highest point on a two-count. As for proper breathing technique, you should inhale on the eccentric and exhale on the concentric. The proper breathing is listed later on prior to each lift explanation just in case.

Lastly, before I get into the workout itself, I have gotten *a lot* of questions from people regarding supplements. For some reason, people today think that if they are not on some sort of supplement, then they are not getting what they can out of working out. For the most part, this is hogwash! It is this belief which makes the supplement industry a multi-billion dollar a year industry. If you are exercising, you will need more intake to keep your body properly fueled. Getting a well-balanced diet is key, as I stated earlier. One recommendation I would make is to increase your protein. Protein is a key factor in muscle growth and development. You can do this by eating more foods with protein in them (clean protein like turkey, chicken, fish…not the fatty proteins found in other sources), or by supplementing with any number of the powders or shakes out on the market. I do not wish to endorse any one type of protein supplement but, if you do choose a protein powder or type of protein bar, I would recommend that it has whey protein as the main source of protein. If it's whey isolate, then that's all the better, but whey concentrate (or a mix of the two) is a good choice also. All that other stuff (creatine, arginine, glutamine, etc.) should be used (if that's what you choose to do) after you have done extensive research on your own, and weighed the pros and cons for yourself.

THE WORKOUT

So here it is. There are many more intricate plans, programs, and so forth, but this one is a great base to build on. All the fancy lifts in the world will do the same thing as these. There may be a day when you move on to those, but for now, let's keep it simple.

The Great 8 Workout

Group One:
Chest
Triceps
Shoulders
Biceps

Group Two:
Lateralis muscles
Quadriceps
Hamstrings
Abdominals

Muscle Groups and Choices:

Group One

Chest:
Bench Press
Incline Bench Press
Dumbbell Flies
Dumbbell Press
"Pec Deck" Fly Machine
Three Stage Pushups
   (Sets of five, ten, or fifteen)

Triceps:
Dips
Throw Backs
Triceps Pull Downs
Close Grip Bench
Nose Breakers
Overhead Triceps

Shoulders:
Military Press
Lateral Raises
Bent Over Flies
Front Raises
Barbell Raises
Wide Grip Upright Rows
Shrugs

Biceps:
Preacher Curls
One-arm Standing Full
   Supination Curls
Hammer Curls
21s
Isolation Curls
Standing Wall Curls
Ten-Second Curls *(sets
   of six reps)*

To Start:

- Pick two exercises for each muscle group.

- For each muscle exercise, start with three sets of ten (certain exercises here will be a little different than 3x10 or 4x10…those will be explained in full).

- Work your way up to three exercises per group; four sets of ten (if you want more challenge as time goes on, make it four exercises, four sets of ten).

- Use the ten reps as a guide for increasing size. If toning is what you want, work up to three or four sets of 12-15 reps (a lighter weight will be needed).

- You should never be longer than sixty minutes in the weight room. Intensity is part of your workout! Minimum one-minute rest between sets maximum two minutes.

Group Two

Lats:
Lawn Mowers
Lat Pull Downs
Straight Arm Pull Downs
Bent Over Rows
Reverse Grip Bent
  Over Rows
Seated Rows

Quads:
Leg Extension
Wall Sits (minimum 1
  minute each)
Dumbbell Squat

Hamstring:
Leg Curls
Straight Leg Dead Lifts
Good Mornings
Flutter Kicks

Leg Combo:
Squats
Plyometric Jumps
  (1 set = 1 Minute)
Lunges
Side Lunges

Abdominals:
Russian Twists
Feet Up Crunch
Leg Lifts
Bicycle Twist Crunch
Side Crunch
Heel Lifts
Leg Climb

To Start:

- Follow along with Group One instructions for working lats.

- For legs, start with one quad, one hamstring, and one leg combo, 2x10. Work your way up to two lifts from each category, 4x10.

- For toning, go with the lighter weight and work 12-15 reps for each set.

- Abdominals—To start, pick as many exercises as you want to do for the day (let's say at least three), and do as many sets necessary to complete 150 abdominal moves total. Over time, you will find that you can do more per set to get to the 150 mark. Eventually, work your rep number up from 150 to 300-350.

HOW IT WORKS

To explain the general formula for how this works (I will get into detailed explanations of what each lift is later), each group should be done twice a week. This is for weight training/resistance type workouts. Cardio is also another consideration (a must for total body change and enhancement).

The first week you begin weight training, you should use (as an example) Monday and Thursday to be your Group One workout days. You want to hit all muscle groups twice a week, but give each group plenty of rest, as well. During that first week, use Tuesday and Friday as your Group Two exercise days. Beginning the second week, flip groups, meaning, Monday and Thursday should be Group Two, and Tuesday and Friday should be Group One. Starting out, begin with two exercises from each list and do three sets of ten repetitions for size, or 12-15 repetitions for toning. As you get more comfortable (probably somewhere around the third week), move this to three lifts from each group, and do four sets of ten (or

12-15, depending on your goals) repetitions. Down the road, if you want a little more challenge, you could go to four lifts per group.

Speaking of beginning, it can be a bit tricky to decide what weight to start with. If you have never lifted weights before, it may take a time or two to figure out where to start. You should start light enough to get the correct form down, but not so light as to get zero benefit (except maybe for bench press and squats, in which starting with the bar to get the form is a good idea; *especially* with these two exercises, *make sure* you have a spotter).

How do you decide at what weight to start with? This is where the trial and error comes into play. First and foremost is proper form. When it comes to sets, you want to challenge yourself with the weight, but make sure it is something that you can accomplish. A good rule to go by is that your last set should be the toughest (obviously)…*if*, as you get rolling, your reps per set go something like ten, ten, eight, seven; I would say that's probably a pretty good weight to work with. Once you can get four sets of ten, if building muscle is what you want, then it's time to move up the weight. The same would hold true for toning, in that if you can get 4 sets of 12-15 reps, move up the weight. As for early on in your program (when you are working on two or three sets of ten), if you get less than eight on your first set, drop the heft of the weight. Now, yes, I did say that each set should consist of ten repetitions. This is the goal. Once you can hit ten (or 12-15) reps with each set, especially your last set, you have accomplished it and should move on up.

Wednesday should be a day to let your body rest, as far as lifting goes. In the beginning, I would recommend taking it off from all exercise, except a warm up and stretch routine. If exercise is brand new to you, I would think the first three or four Wednesdays should be a good day to just get a good stretch (both groups 1 and 2 stretches) and otherwise use as a recovery day. As far as exercise, Wednesday would be a good day to work on things like agility training, coordination drills, or cardio, which you could do during lifting days, as well if you choose to.

STARTING EACH WORKOUT

Before I get into each lift, let's talk a little about warming up and cooling down. As for warming up, one should never just jump into the weight room and start hitting the weights. This is a great way to pull, tear, or otherwise hurt muscles, which usually turns people off from restarting. So, in order to do it right, I recommend something like this (it would take about five minutes or so to get your body ready). Since a muscle is more pliable (stretchy) when it is warm, start with something like a two minute jog (run in place if you don't have the room), fifty to a hundred jumping jacks, or something similar to get the blood flowing.

Then, for each muscle group you are going to work, take about a minute per each to stretch (if it is a group one day work out, stretch all the major muscle groups listed in the group one workout, same for group two). I will put in some stretches to give you some examples later. After a workout, it is extremely important to stretch each muscle group worked. This will help with getting blood flow to these areas you worked to help begin the rebuilding process, and will also help you keep your flexibility.

Stretching before and after a workout can help you reach your goals sooner. Stretching can also help increase and/or keep your flexibility (remember that comment earlier about muscle bound?). The stretches in here are, for the most part, static stretches, meaning that you hold each stretch and then relax. I like to hold each stretch for about twenty to thirty seconds, and then relax it, and stretch the same muscle again. If you do this right, the second time through you should be stretching a little farther than the first time. This is good, as you are getting deeper into the muscle fibers.

Very important: do not bounce your stretches. There is a form of stretching known as ballistic stretching, which can be good during a routine, but for our purposes let's stick to the static pre and post workout stuff. Bouncing (or overstretching) can lead to injury and that (obviously) would be bad and not what we are out for here.

So how do you know when you stretched far enough? Your body will let you know. It should be a little uncomfortable, but not horrifically painful. Strive for each stretch to be a little farther than the previous. It is very important that you *do not bounce!* You are trying to prepare your muscles for work, not injury. Over time, you will notice that stretching comes much easier and your flexibility will increase. This will help you with many facets of life, as well as improving overall health.

LET'S DO THIS!

Okay, so here we go. I am going to break down each group by category and explain the proper techniques to keep in mind for each. If you are just starting, if this is your first ever lift, *do not get stuck on how much you can (or cannot) lift!* Technique here is *way* more important than that. For some of these, just the bar will be fine until you get the proper form down.

I think it is worthy to mention here that, as you get into reading how to perform each lift, it may not be the most exciting thing you have ever read. Still, I implore you to read through each exercise, especially if you are not familiar with lifting or any of these lifts. It would be better to make sure you have the technique right than find out the hard way, which might lead to injury.

Group One Stretches

The first part of every workout is the warm up. I will, from here on out, assume that you got the blood moving to warm up the muscles that are going to be worked today, whether it was a little jogging or running in place, some jumping jacks, or whatever you do to get a little sweat going. Do the warm up and all the stretches for the day at the beginning. It is not necessary to do a separate warm up and stretch when you move from one muscle group to the other.

In general, the warm up should take about five to no more than ten minutes, and all groups to be worked for the day should be ready to go. Just as important, you should also properly cool down when you are finished. A proper cool down would include everything as far as the stretches listed go (no need to run in place or anything like that). This will help you maintain that flexibility we have talked about, as well as aid your muscles in recovering from the day's work. Lastly, as you stretch (for both Group One and Group Two), remember to breathe, breathe, breathe! Slow, even inhales, followed by slow and even exhales. It's hard to imagine, but some folks tend to hold their breath while they stretch, or even sort of pant like a dog. Stretching should be somewhat relaxing, and the breathing will get the oxygen flowing through the muscles either getting them ready to work or helping to relax them afterwards. I have also found the pre-workout stretch a great opportunity to clear the mind and focus on the upcoming task at hand (the workout). The post-workout stretch is a good chance to calmly reflect on how things went.

Some good stretches to do here are as follows. You can also check out the example pictures, to clear up any confusion. Do not skip this part! Not only should you keep reading, but you *definitely* don't want to skip the warm up and stretch before working out. As I have mentioned before, you should also go through the stretch part of this at the end, to help your muscles recover and to aid in the cool down.

Neck Stretch (stretches the neck and upper shoulder muscles)

Stand with your feet shoulder width apart, arms straight, palms out. Gently lean your head to the right, trying to touch your right ear to your right shoulder. Hold for about five to ten seconds, then slowly roll your head to the left (as you roll, try to touch your chin to your chest) and repeat the stretch on the other side. Stretch each side about three times. As you do this stretch, reach your hands to the ground so you don't shrug.

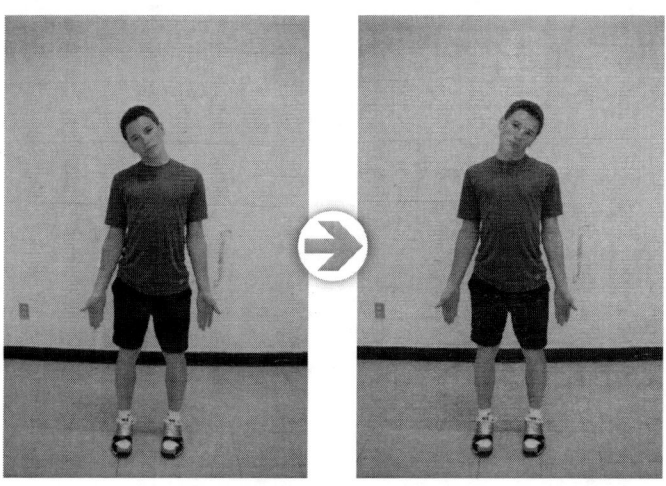

Sky Scraper (stretches the chest muscles)

Stand up tall; feet shoulder width apart with a slight bend in the knees. Take both arms and extend them above your head as high as you can reach. Bend your elbows so you form a ninety-degree angle. While doing this, slowly begin to lower the upper part of your arms. Lower your elbows, and pretend that you are trying to scrape an imaginary wall behind you (or pretend you are trying to touch your elbows together behind your back). Do this about three to four times. Remember to *slowly* bring your elbows down.

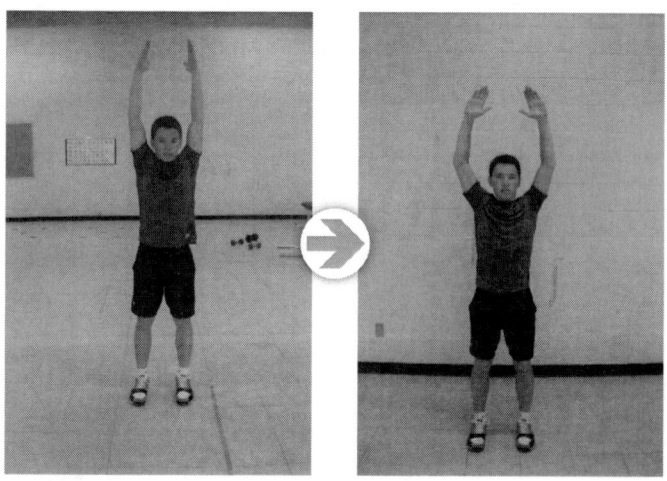

Wall Stretch (stretches the chest as well as the biceps muscles)

Stand facing a wall, placing one arm up parallel to the ground. Keep your arm straight, palm on the wall, and *slowly* twist your body in the opposite direction of your parallel arm until it feels a little uncomfortable. Hold for about twenty to thirty seconds for each arm. Keep as much of your arm from palm to shoulder on the wall.

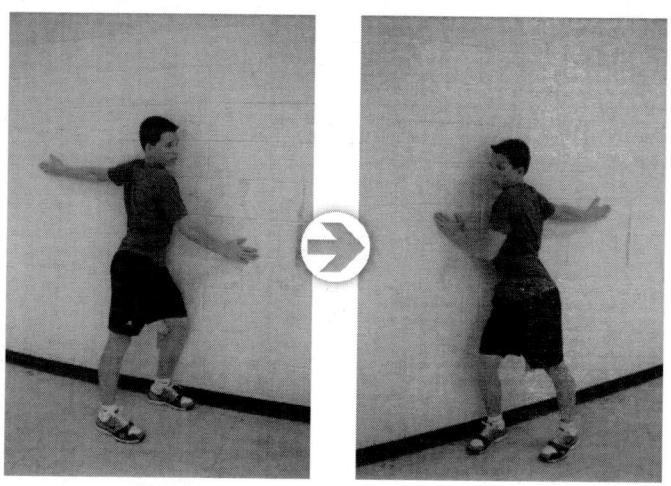

Trunk Twist (stretches the chest, oblique, and even in your abdominal muscles)

Take a light, straight bar and place it on your shoulders. Keep your arms wide, palms facing away from you, and slowly rotate your trunk from side to side. Hold each rotation for about five seconds. Get about three to five twists per side.

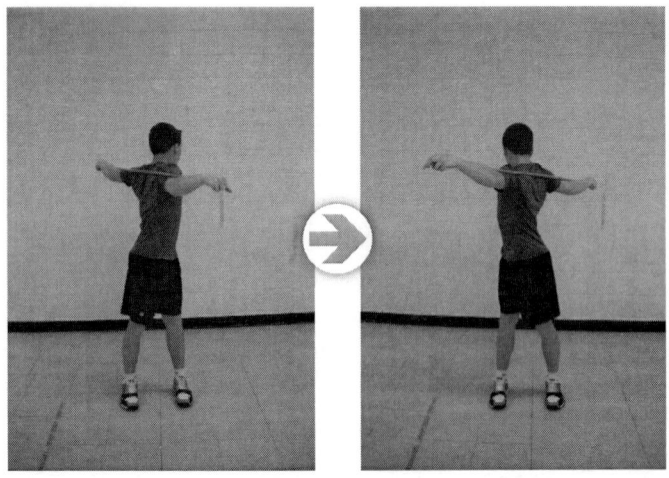

Overhead Bent Arm (stretches the triceps muscles)

Take one arm and extend it above your head. Bend the elbow behind your head, palm facing the back of your neck. Grasp either your wrist or elbow (if you are that flexible) and pull your arm until you feel the stretch in your triceps. Hold for 20-30 seconds, then repeat on the other arm. Do each arm twice.

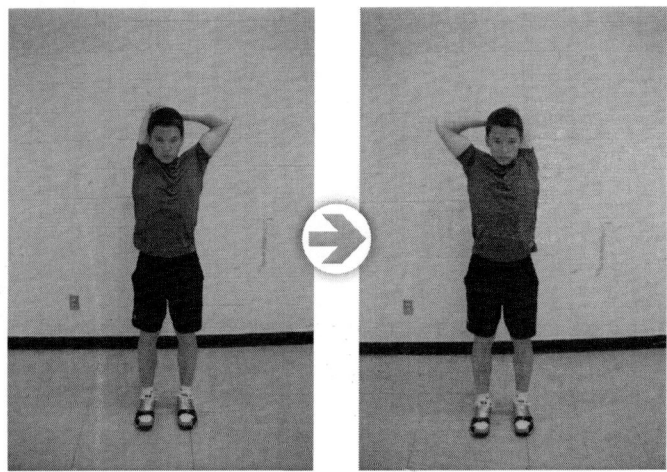

Static Hugger (stretches the shoulder and upper back muscles)

Take one arm at a time, and place it across your body, just under your chin. With your other arm, hook the upper part of your arm just above the elbow and gently pull. Hold for about ten to thirty seconds. Do both arms twice.

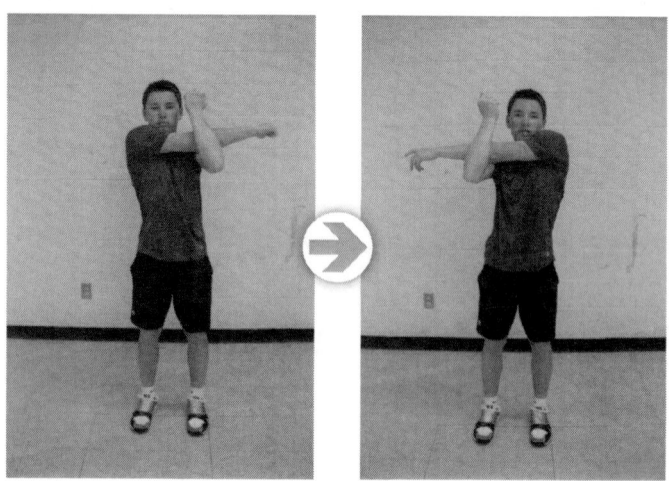

Straight Arm Clasp (stretches the shoulder and upper back muscles)

Put your arms straight down in front of you and cross your wrists, placing the palms together. Try to roll the shoulders to touch in the front. Hold for about ten to thirty seconds.

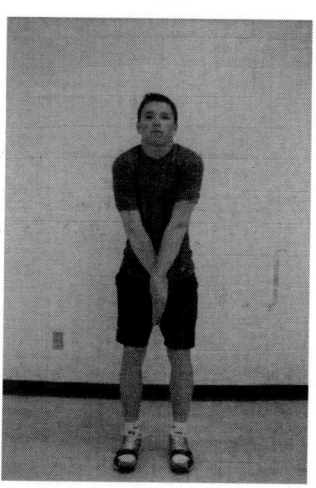

Reverse Straight Arm Clasp (stretches the shoulder, biceps, and chest muscles)

Clasp your hands behind you, elbows bent (to start) in the small of your back. Straighten your arms and roll your shoulders back so that you stand up straight, chest out, as if you are trying to touch your shoulder blades together. Hold for ten to thirty seconds.

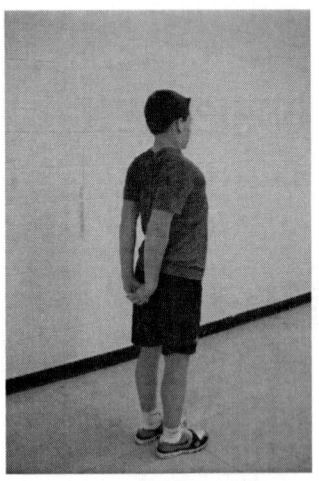

Unless otherwise noted, the exercises fit the two to four sets of ten (or 12-15) rule discussed earlier. Now you are ready to hit the weight pile.

Chest

(Breathing: Inhale as the weight moves towards you, exhale as the weight moves away from you)

Bench Press

First and foremost, you *definitely* need a spotter for this exercise. If, for some reason, you are alone, do *not* bench press! Just as important as a spotter, keep your back on the bench and your feet on the floor. Many people, when first starting to bench press, either kick their feet all over, or arch their back off of the bench. By keeping your feet on the floor, you will maintain your balance and keep your leverage. Arching your back can lead to injury.

As you lie down, make sure that the bar is right about eye level as you look up at it. Hands should be evenly spaced, a little farther than shoulder width apart. As you lift the bar off of the holder, keep it steady above your chest. This is where the four count-two count comes into play. Bring the weight (or bar, for starters) down to your chest (aim for the middle of your breast bone) on a four count and explode up on a two count.

This may sound like a no brainer, but I have seen it happen too many times not to mention this. *Do not* bounce the weight off your chest! Control the weight to your body *(*hence the four count*)*. As for hitting your chest, it is not totally required to touch your chest with the weight. Controlling the weight down until your upper arms are slightly less than parallel with the floor will suffice. For obvious reasons, using your chest as a sling shot will not make you stronger, tougher, or better at bench press. What it will do (potentially) for you is crack some ribs, cause injury, turn you off from lifting, or keep you out of the weight room.

Keep your head for this and pretty much all lifts in a neutral position, which is to say that your neck is straight, your chin is up, and your eyes are looking straight ahead, no matter what position your body is in.

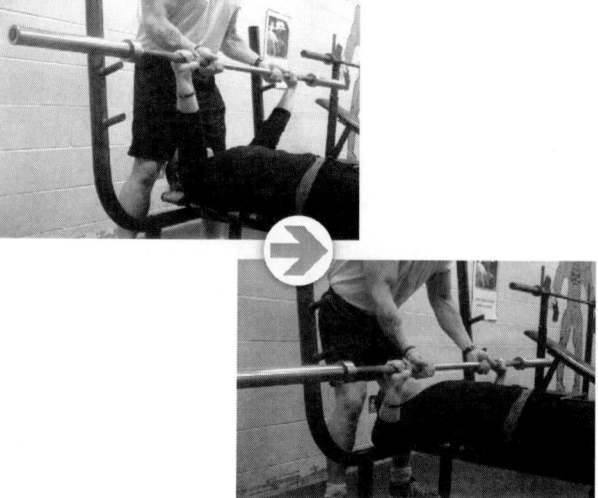

Incline Bench Press

As for grip, the distance between your hands here is the same as bench press. One thing you will find is that you won't be able to do as much weight as a regular flat bench press. This lift isolates the upper portion of your chest muscles (your pectoral muscles, for those of you who like a more technical name), so you will be using less of the total muscle to do this.

Guide the weight down to your chest on a four count. This time, aim for the upper portion of your chest, just below the collarbone. Make sure you aim right, and not on your face or neck. It would seem like a no brainer, but it is amazing what people will do.

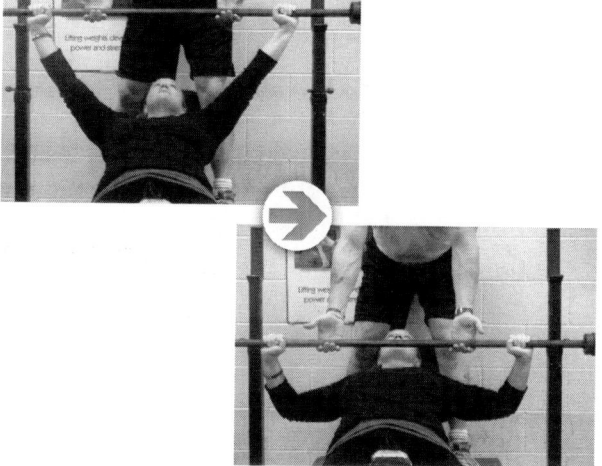

Dumbbell Flies

For this move, make sure that your feet are planted and your back stays on the bench. When first doing this, you will notice that to stay balanced is a little more difficult than a bench press.

Make sure to keep your elbow slightly bent throughout this move, to take any unnecessary strain off of your elbow joint. This is something I call hugging the barrel. There are other moves that will be explained where you should keep a slight bend in the elbow throughout the exercise.

Start with the weights above you, palms facing each other, weights touching (photo 1). Going on the four count, bring your hands apart, maintaining that barrel hug throughout until your upper arms are just below parallel to the floor (photo 2). Control it down, of course. From here, bring the weights back together.

When you finish your set, it is very important to keep control of the weights. Many times, people will just drop them, and they can bounce and cause damage to property and people. I find it best to lay them on my upper thighs (while still lying down), and sit up with them in my lap (photos 3 and 4). A lot safer for all involved.

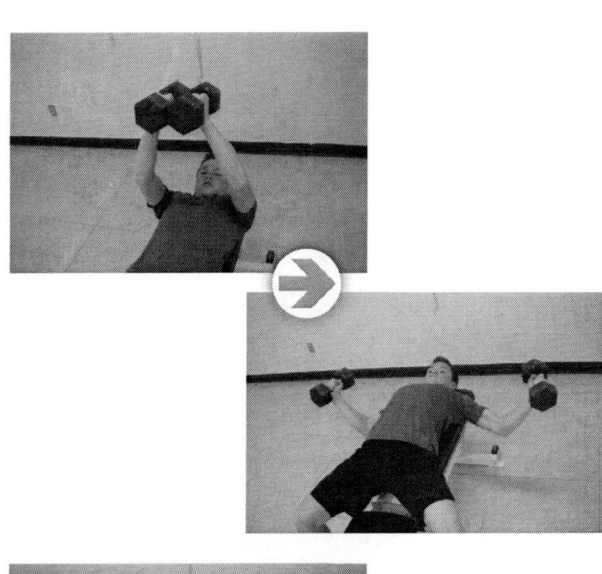

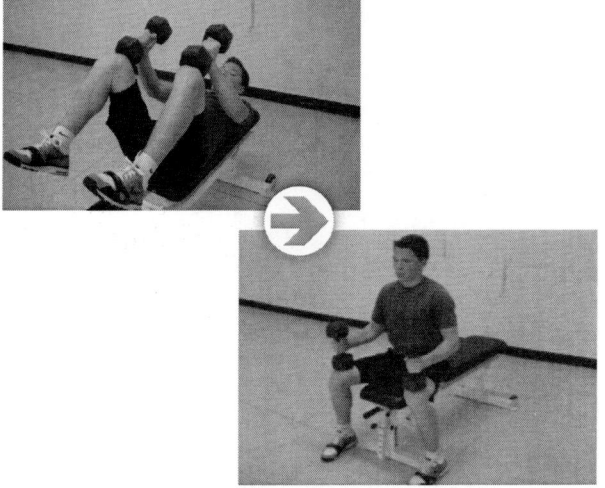

WHAT ARE YOU WAITING FOR?

Dumbbell Press

As before, keep the feet planted and the back flat. There are a couple of different variations as to how to do this exercise. One would be the wide grip press, in which you keep your hands wide apart throughout the entire move as if you were holding a bar bell doing a regular bench press.

The other technique would be to start with the weights together, palms facing each other (just like the starting position for dumbbell flies). As you bring your arms down, widen your hands apart and rotate your wrists out. Your hands should be wide apart, as if you were holding a barbell, at the bottom of this move. As you bring your arms up, rotate the palms together again. You could mix these two techniques up any way you wish. Some people find one or the other version more of a challenge. As with the dumbbell flies, control the weight down until your upper arms are just past parallel to the floor. Make sure also that when you finish, you use the sit up method, and don't just drop them.

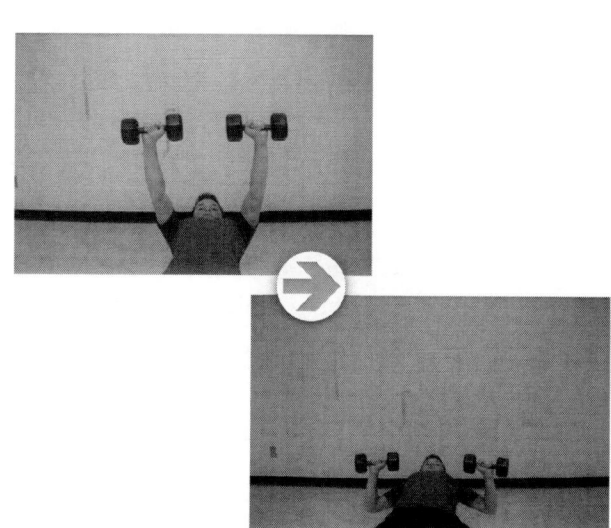

Pec Deck Fly Machine

If possible, you want to set this machine up so that your feet are on the ground and your back is flat against the back of the chair. If the machine has the pads (like the one shown), put the chair at a height where your upper arms are parallel with the floor. Depending on your height and the height of the machine, you may or may not be able to get your feet on the floor. It is more important that your arms are parallel if you have to make a choice.

This exercise starts with your forearms together (photo 1). To get properly set up, pull your arms in front of you one at a time. If you attempt to pull both arms at once, you could over stress your joints. This would be bad.

Once you are set up with the pads in front of you, control the weight back using the four-count method until your upper arms are almost straight across your body (photo 2). Don't let them get behind your chest, as this could add undo and unwanted strain on your shoulders, and could lead to injury. To finish the move, bring both arms together again, simultaneously using the two count. As with starting the exercise, when you finish, control one arm back at a time to release the weight (photos 3 and 4).

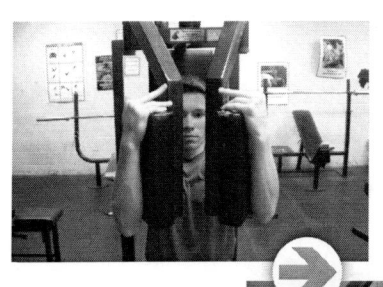

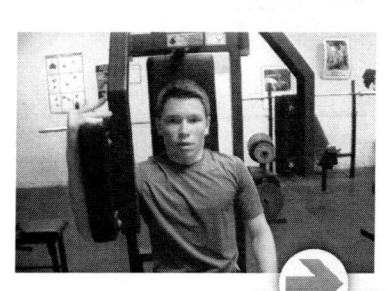

WHAT ARE YOU WAITING FOR?

Three Stage Pushups

(Sets of five, ten, or fifteen)

This goes against the ten-rep rule. You can, however, do the two to four sets. The way this works is that each set will be fifteen, thirty, or forty-five pushups in a row. I will explain using the set of five.

Start with doing five reps of a regular width push up, which is to say that your hands are directly under your shoulders (pictures 1 and 2). Immediately after the first five, widen your hands and do five wide arm pushups. A good distance here is to widen your thumb out to just past where your pinky was during the normal pushup (pictures 3 and 4). After five wide arm pushups, do five diamond pushups, in which your index fingers and thumbs are touching (pictures 5 and 6). For these last five make sure that your upper arms stay tight to your body. It is best if your elbows rub your rib cage as you go down. For the diamond pushups, you may widen your feet if you wish. Feet together (as shown) or wide, either way is fine. For all pushups, you should be exhaling as you push away from the floor.

The proper form for a push up is to keep your back straight at all times. Make sure you maintain a neutral spine with feet together, and you should bend the elbows until they are roughly ninety-degrees. The only part of your body that should bend is your arms. The rest of you should be straight like a 2x4. As you advance with these, you could move up to the tens or fifteens, or even more if you wish.

If necessary, you could start these (or even finish) with your knees on the ground. I know there is a stigma about knees on the ground being for girls only, but if you are spent, it's a good way to get the reps in and still be working. I am not ashamed to admit that there are times when I have done so many pushups that I couldn't finish the normal way, and had to drop my knees to the ground to get the reps in. One final thought here to add a little challenge down the road would be to use push up bars for the regular and wide width pushups to increase your range of motion.

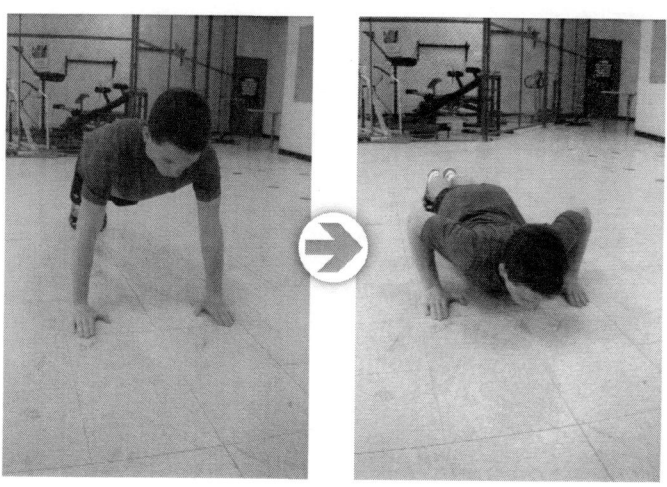

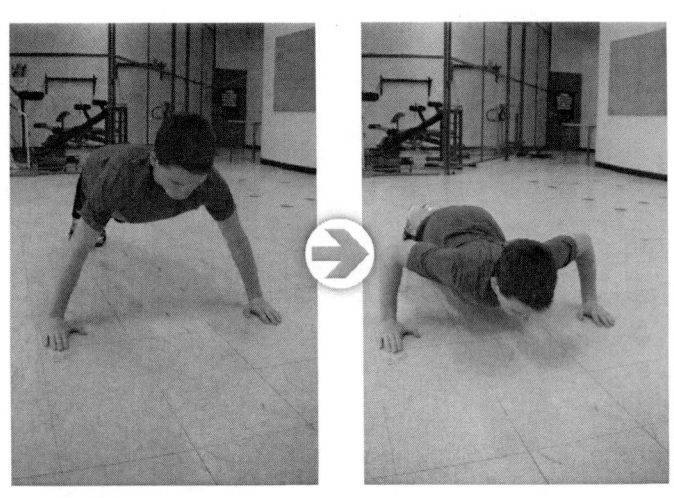

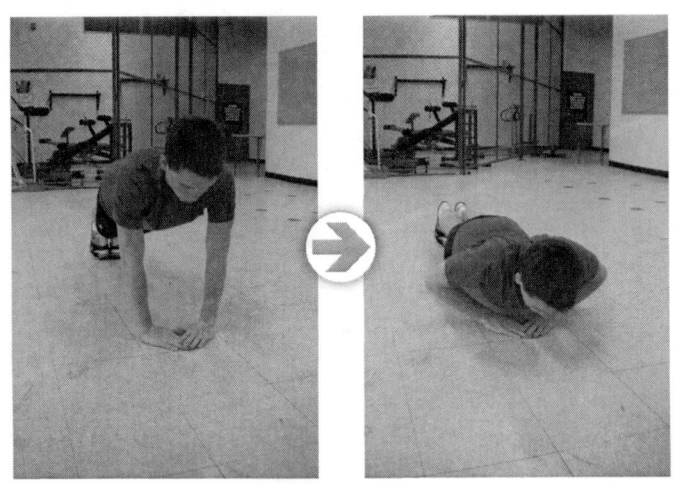

Triceps

(Breathing: Inhale when you bend your elbow(s), exhale as you straighten your arms)

Dips

This exercise can fit the two to four sets of ten (or 12-15), or if you feel up to it, it can become (as time goes on and you get more proficient at lifting) two to four sets of going to failure (which means doing as many as possible until you cannot do any more for that set).

In order to do a proper dip, begin with straight arms and your elbows locked. During this exercise, keep your elbows in tight to your sides. This will help isolate the triceps muscles, and also reduce the risk of injury. You can use a chair or some other helper to get into position. It would also be a good idea to keep the chair nearby as you get started, so you could use it as an assist if you need to. From the up position, slowly control your body downward until your elbows are at ninety-degrees. Then, push your way back up to the straight-arm position. Make sure that the only part of your body that is moving is your arms. Keep your lower half from wiggling around. It is okay to keep your legs straight or cross them and bend at the knee.

A word of encouragement: In the beginning, these can be a lot tougher than they look. Stick with it. If you have difficulty, you can use the chair to hold part of your weight on (like one foot or to partially push up with) as you work. Another good way to develop the skill for this is to work the eccentric phase only at first and use your assister to get back to the start position. Over time, work your way into at least 3-4 sets of ten.

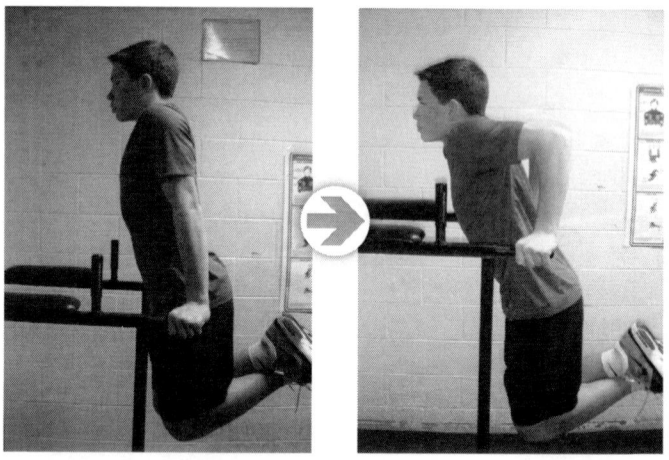

Throw Backs

As you begin this exercise, make sure that you maintain a good, flat back throughout the entire movement. Another key point here is that you need to keep your elbow in contact with your rib cage throughout the entire movement. Otherwise, you are working more than just the triceps and defeating the purpose of this exercise.

Start with your elbow at ninety-degrees , forearm towards the floor. As the exercise indicates, throw the weight back so that your arm is straight. Control the weight back to the starting position.

It's not that uncommon to find that one arm has a harder time with the same weight. If you find that you have a weaker arm, work that arm first, so you know how many to do on the other side. Over time, your weak arm will catch up.

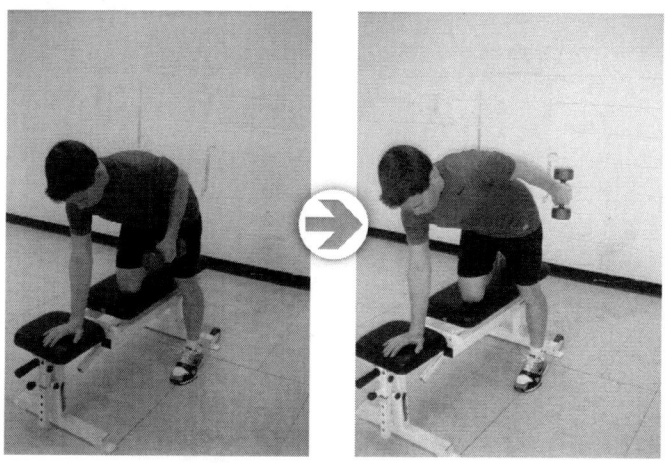

Triceps Push Downs

First off, make sure you have a good base for this exercise. By that, I mean that your feet are shoulder width apart, knees slightly bent, back straight, and, of course, the head in the neutral position. Start with the bar by your waist. I find it easiest to take a step back with one foot and pull the bar to my midsection to help get set up. Keep your hands about shoulder width apart (you could go a little closer if you wish).

Throughout this exercise, your elbows should stay in contact with your ribs. This is very important. Allowing your arms to swing around will not isolate the triceps properly. As you begin, slowly bend your elbows until they hit the ninety-degree mark. Then, push the weight back down to your waist. The way I think of this is the movement is from beltline to belly button.

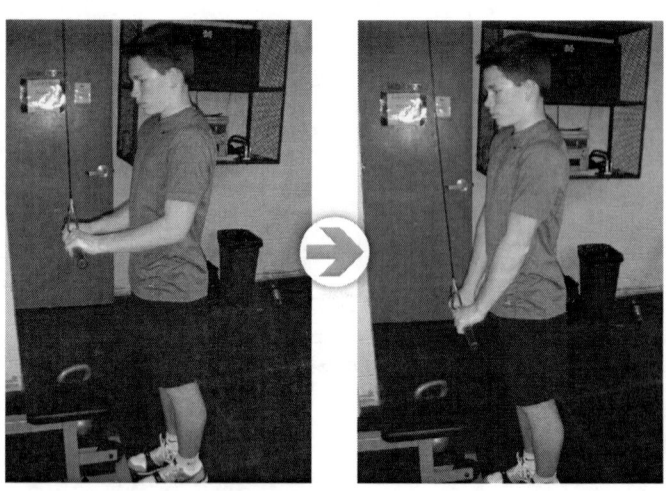

Close Grip Bench Press

The difference between this and a regular Bench Press is that your hands should be close enough that your elbows and forearms rub your rib cage on each repetition. Any closer than the width of your ribs and you will put undo strain on your wrists.

It may seem an obvious point here, but you will not be able to use the same weight as you did for your regular bench press. By bringing your arms in close, you are isolating the triceps more, so you will need to decrease the amount you lift. It may take a time or two to get this figured out, but it is a very worthwhile lift. Your aiming point will be a little lower than the normal bench press. Control the weight down to the lower part of your ribs, and then push back up to the starting point.

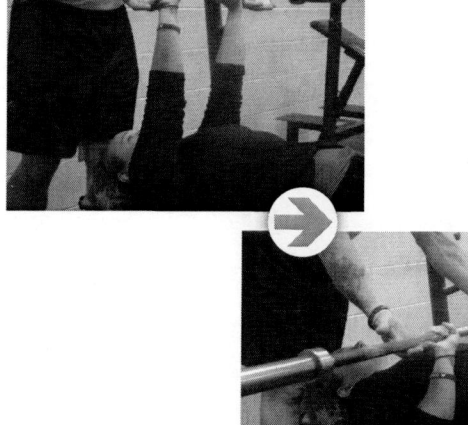

Nose Breakers

As far as form, it is very similar to bench press, in that your feet and back should stay stationary. It would be worth mentioning early that for this exercise, do *not* try to force extra reps. If you feel yourself faltering, you are done. Fighting for extra reps here might wind up with you dropping the weight on your face.

Start with the weight above your chest, arms straight. Slowly control the weight down towards your head, until your reach about the ninety-degree mark. It is very important to keep your upper arms completely still during this move. The only thing that should be moving is the joint in your elbow. As with the dumbbell flies and press, when you have completed your set, *gently* place the weight on your mid-section and do a sit up.

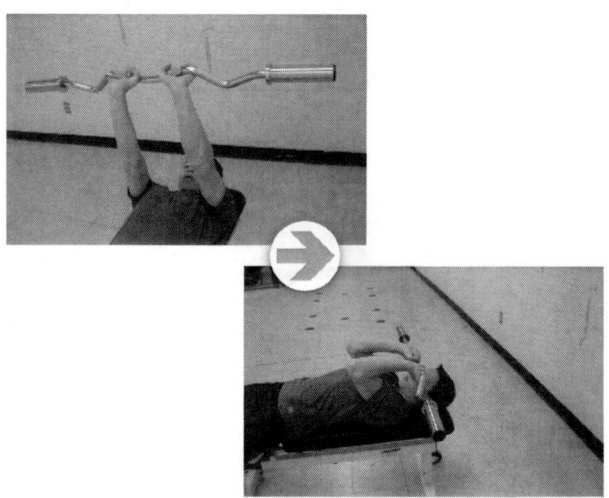

Overhead Triceps

As with the nose breakers, this is a move where you don't want to struggle to get one more rep. To start, make sure your feet are planted and stay firmly on the ground. I would recommend, at least until you gain some experience, that you use a chair (or bench) that has a back to it, so that you don't arch and also to help you maintain good form.

As you can see, your head should remain in the neutral position throughout the exercise. Keep the weight firmly locked in your palms between your thumbs and forefingers. Your upper arms should maintain constant contact with the side of your head. By making sure your upper arms are touching the side of your head, you will guarantee good form. This is also one of those exercises where the only movement should come from the bending of the elbow joint.

As discussed before, guide and control the weight until your elbows are at the ninety-degree point, and then push it back up. Starting out, a couple of things to keep in mind are that you should use a lighter weight to make sure you get the proper form, and if getting to ninety-degrees is hard, work your way up to it. Bring the weight down until you hit that point of no return and then push back up. Over time, increase the elbow bend until you reach ninety degrees.

As with other exercises already discussed, when you are finished with your set, bring the weight to your lap instead of dropping it behind you.

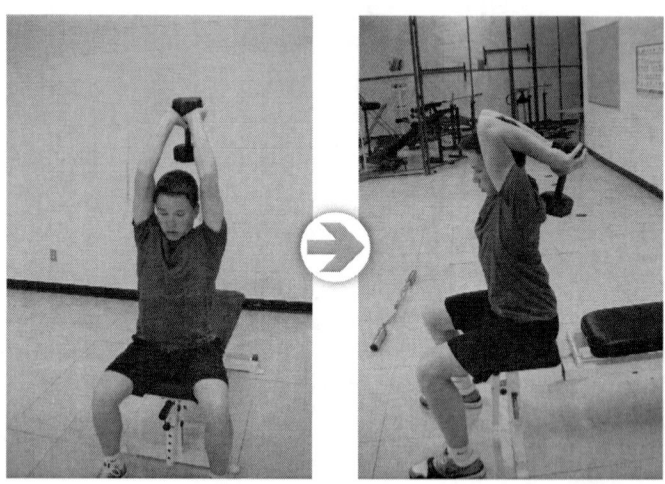

Shoulders

(Breathing: Inhale the weight towards you, exhale as the weight moves away from you)

Military Press

Start with the seat back straight up, forming a ninety degree angle. You could do this with either a couple of dumbbells or a barbell. Try it with both techniques to see what feels more comfortable to you. If you choose the barbell, it is very important that you never bring the weight for this exercise behind your head. Dumbbells might, at first, be a little harder to balance, so you should start with a light weight. Keep the feet firmly planted on the floor and your back against the chair.

Start with the weight above you, arms extended. Control the weight down until your upper arms are slightly less than parallel to the floor (similar to Bench Pressing), then push the weight back up. Keep the weight in front of you, and never behind you. This is important to help reduce injury to your shoulders and upper back and neck area. If you have an opportunity, set up for this lift in front of a mirror. That way, you will be able to keep your head in the neutral position, but be able to monitor proper form, as well as make sure you are bringing the weight down to the proper angle.

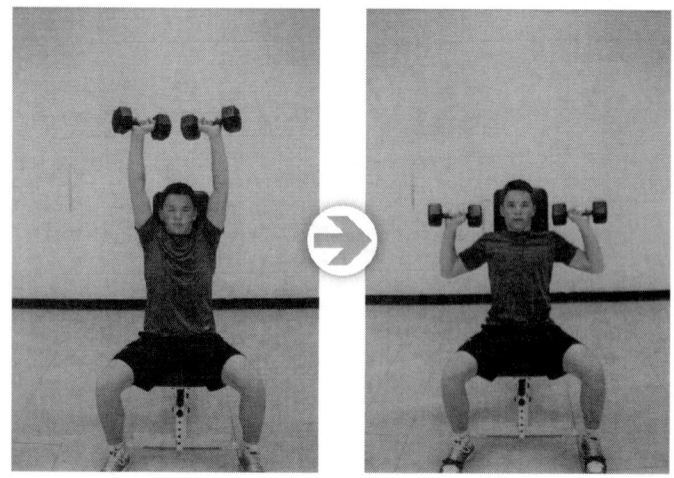

Lateral Raises

Start with the weights at your side, legs shoulder width apart, and a slight bend in the knees. From here, raise your arms up to the side so that your arms become parallel with the ground and your upper body forms a "T". Keep a *slight* bend in the elbow to keep the strain off of the elbow joint. Slowly control the weight back to your side.

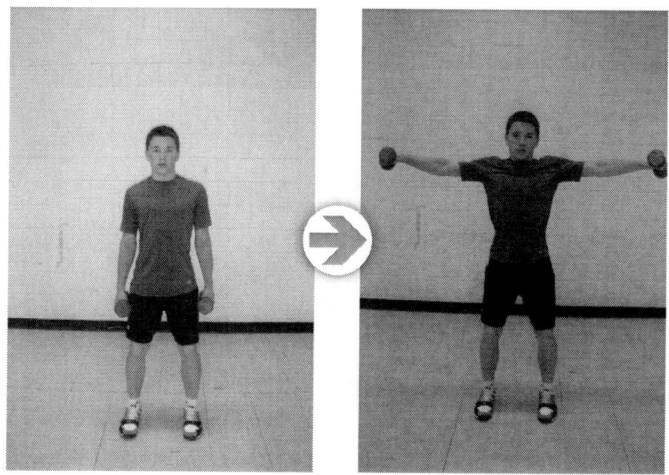

Bent Over Flies

For this exercise, stand with your feet wider than shoulder width and a slight bend in the knee. Bend from the waist so that your back is parallel with the floor. Keep your elbows bent at about a forty-five-degree angle throughout the exercise. As mentioned earlier, this is the hugging a barrel form. With palms facing each other, pull your arms upward toward the ceiling until your upper arms are parallel with the floor. Slowly guide the weight back down. Be sure that, as your elbows come up, and that you keep them straight so as to create that "T" with your upper body. Do not allow them to float back towards your lower back and/or hips.

It is very important to maintain that neutral position with your head. Make sure throughout this exercise you are staring at the floor. No need to strain your neck. If you find that doing this becomes stressful on your lower back, you can also modify this move and sit in a chair. What you would want to do is sit on the edge of the chair, and lean forward until the bottom of your rib cage touches your thighs. The arm movement is the same.

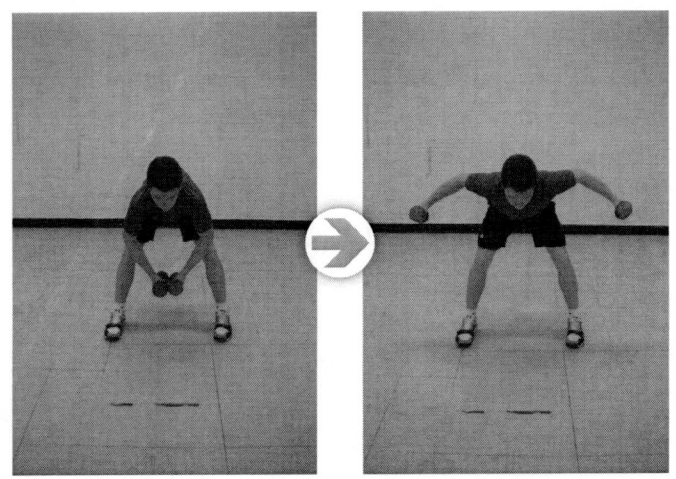

Front Raises

We are back to a more normal stance, feet shoulder width apart, knees slightly bent. Start with your hands down, palms against the thighs. Raise one arm at a time until your forearm is parallel with the ground. Control the weight to the start position. Alternate arms, but do one complete repetition before starting on the other arm. Be conscious of keeping a good, straight, and stationary back as you lift each arm. Do not arch the weight up. Lastly, for this exercise, doing one rep with each arm should count as one, not two reps (a set of 10 would be 10 for each arm, not 10 total).

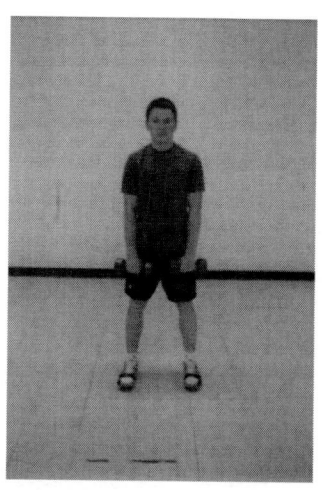
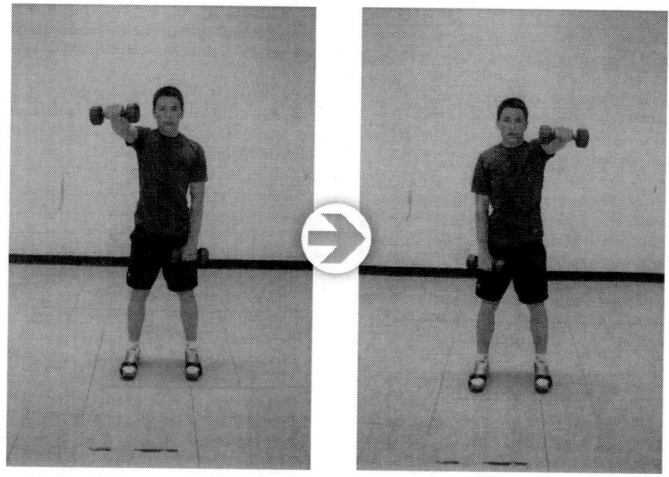

WHAT ARE YOU WAITING FOR?

Barbell Raises

This is the same move as the Front Raise, except now you will have to lighten the load to maintain good form. You could use a straight barbell, or you may find it easier to use a curl bar for this. As for hands, you can play with the distance between them, from shoulder width to a little wider. Don't go closer than shoulder width though, as it may cause unnecessary strain on your wrists. Raise the barbell until your arms are parallel with the floor, and then guide the weight back down to the starting position.

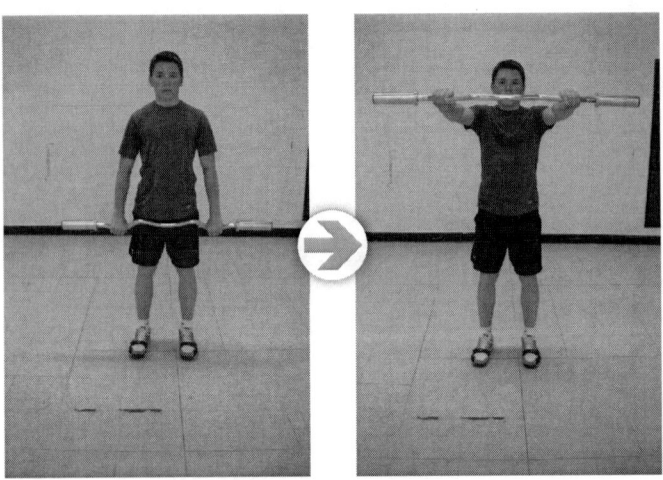

Wide Grip Upright Rows

Wide grip means wider than your shoulders. The stance for this is the same as the Front Raises described above. You can use either a barbell or a pair of dumbbells, whichever you feel more comfortable with.

Starting with the bar at your waistline and your arms straight, raise the bar to a point between your upper chest and just beneath your chin. Allow your elbows to flare out away from your body. At the top of the lift, your elbows should be higher than your wrists. Keep your torso from moving (no arching!). Once you reach the top of the lift, slowly guide the weight back to the starting position.

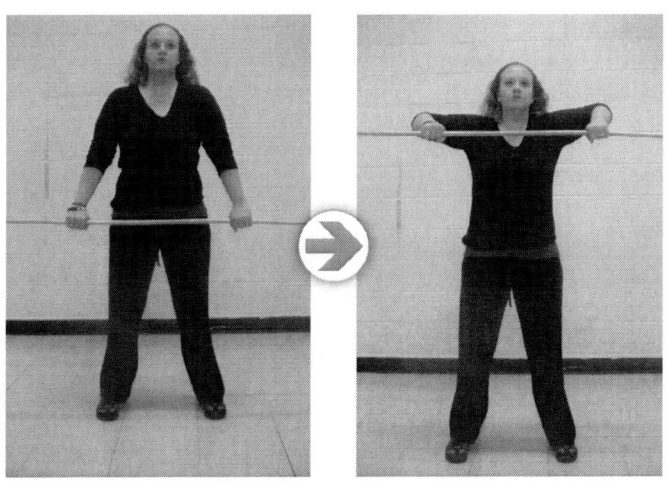

Shrugs

The stance is the same as before, with your feet shoulder width apart, and a slight bend in the knee. Make sure throughout this whole exercise that the only movement you have comes from the shoulder.

Keep the weights steady in your hands with your arms hanging straight down throughout the entire exercise. This is a nice, slow, four count move. The first part is to roll your shoulders forward (photo 1). Shrug upwards as if you are trying to touch your ears with your shoulders (photo 2). Slowly rotate your shoulders backwards, like you are attempting to touch your shoulder blades together (photo 3), and lastly, return to the relaxed pre lift stance (photo 4). You can and should vary this movement by doing an equal number of sets starting the four count rolling your shoulders forward and backward (ex. If you do a set of ten, do five rolling forward first, and five rolling backwards trying to touch your shoulder blades together first).

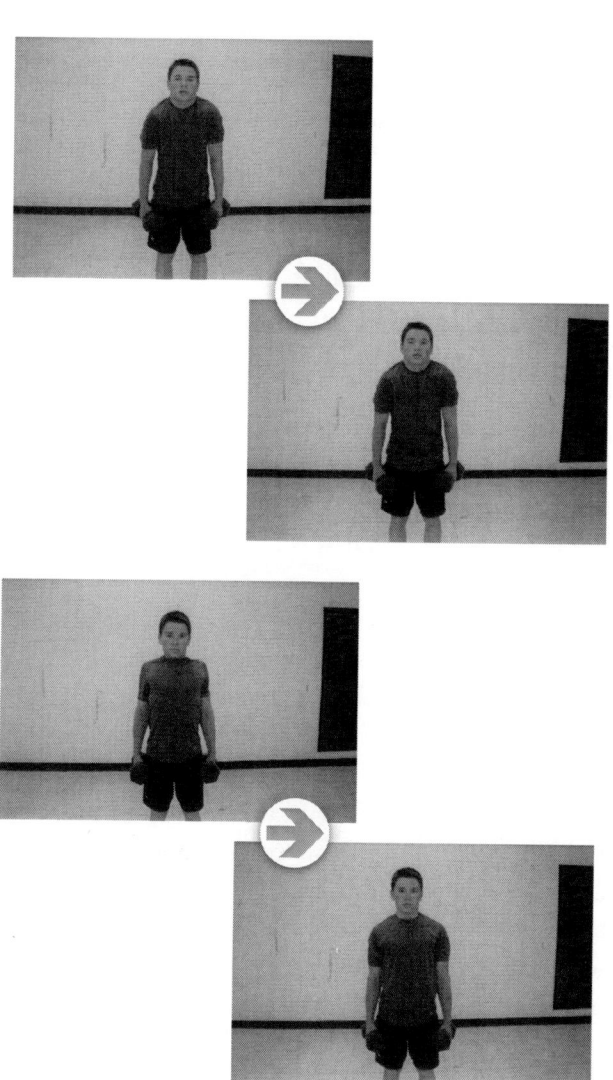

Biceps

(Breathing: Exhale as the weight comes towards you, inhale as it goes away from you)

Please note: As a general rule, for all curls in which you are standing, keep the elbows in contact with your body at all times throughout the lift!

Preacher Curls

Make sure that you set the seat part of the apparatus so that your feet are flat on the ground and the upper portion should be set so that it is tight in your armpits with about a forty-five-degree angle in your shoulder/ upper arm.

It may feel a little awkward at first, but you will get the hang of it. Before sitting down, position yourself above the chair and pick the weight up first. Sit after you have picked up the weight so as to not strain the elbow joint. Start this exercise with the weight under your chin. Control the weight down so that there is a little more than a ninety-degree bend away from you in your elbow. From this point, return the weight back to under your chin to complete the rep. Don't let your arms straighten. This could put too much stress on the elbow possibly causing injury. Lastly, upon completion of your set, hold the weight near your chin until you stand up, and then place it back on the rack, the same way you picked it up.

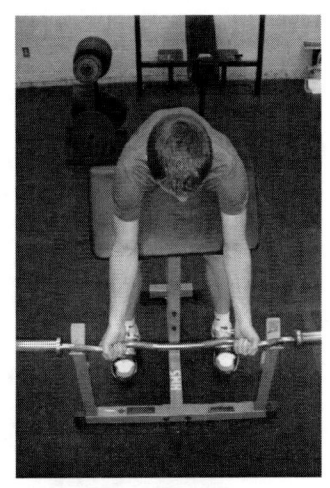

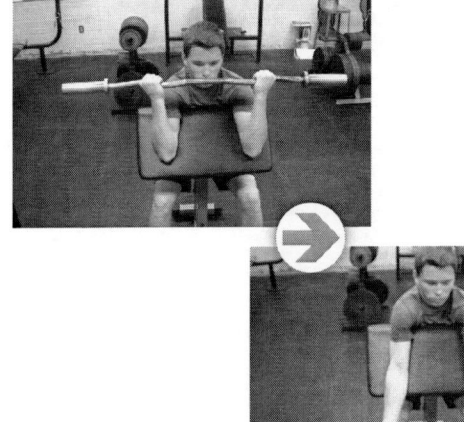

One-Arm Standing Full Supination Curls

The stance for this is the same as discussed previously. Start with the weight at your sides, palms in towards your thighs. One arm at a time, bring the weight from your hip to your shoulder, rotating the weight towards your face as you bring it up (this rotation means full supination. A fancy name for a simple twist of the wrist). As you bring the weight to your shoulder, continue rotating the weight outwards, putting a good squeeze into your bicep. Alternate repetitions, but make sure you complete each individual lift before starting on the other arm (just like the front raises). A set of ten here means ten for each arm, not ten total (meaning only five for each arm). Lastly, keep your back straight and your elbows tight on your sides and don't swing the weight.

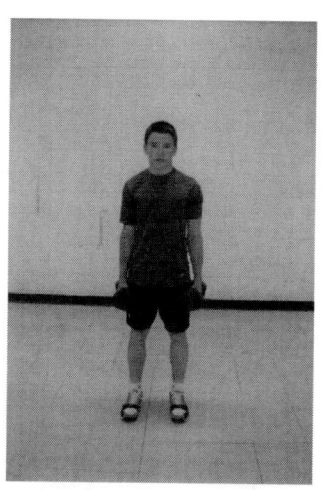
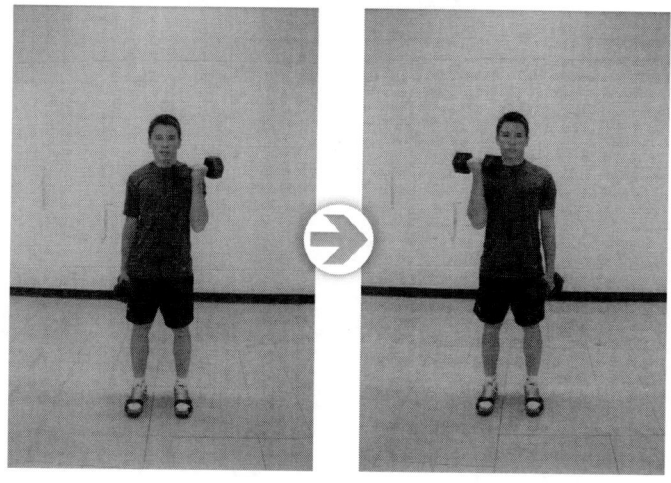

Hammer Curls

This one is exactly as described in the one-arm standing full supination curls. The only difference here is that you don't rotate your wrist on the way up. Keep your wrist turned as if you were hitting a nail throughout the entire movement. As with the full supination curls, fully complete a rep before starting a rep on the other arm.

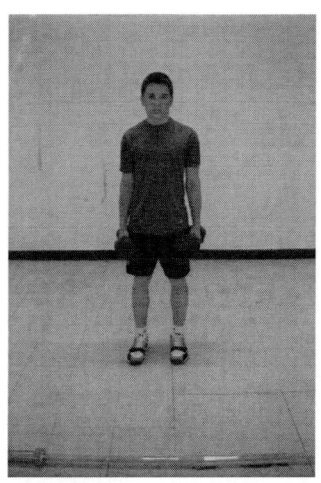

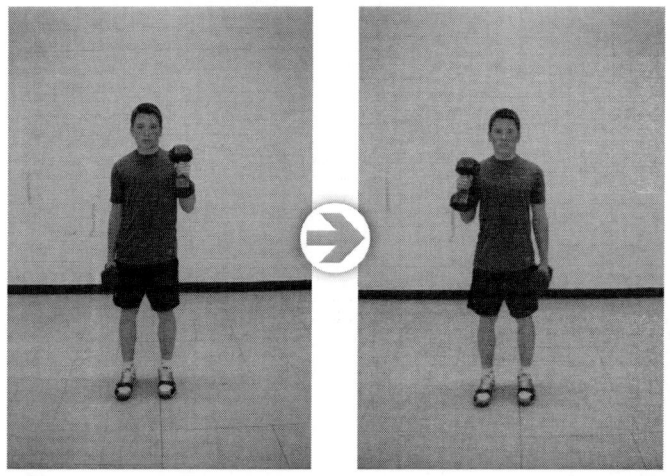

21s

(Does *not* fit the two to four sets of ten)

First, one complete set equals twenty-one reps. Starting this exercise is the same as the One-Arm Standing Full Supination Curl, except that you will do both arms at the same time. Also, these are non-supinated, meaning that you should keep your wrists and palms facing up. No rotating.

To begin, you will start with your arms at your sides. The first portion of this consists of seven lower half curls (pictures 1 and 2). Bring your arms from your waist up until your elbows are ninety-degrees and then back to the starting position. The second portion of this exercise consists of seven upper half curls (pictures 3 and 4). Starting with your elbows bent to ninety-degrees, bring your arms up as close to your shoulders as possible, and then return to the ninety-degree start. The last seven will be the more traditional standing curl (pictures 5 and 6). This is a lot. If you don't manage to get all twenty-one your first time out, don't fret. Stick with it. Lastly, don't sacrifice form to finish. If you start to lose your form, take a break, put the weight down, or stop all together. Poor form can lead to injury.

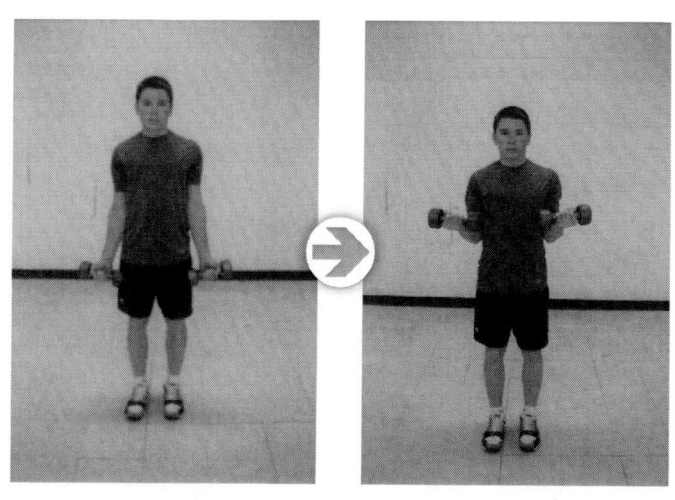

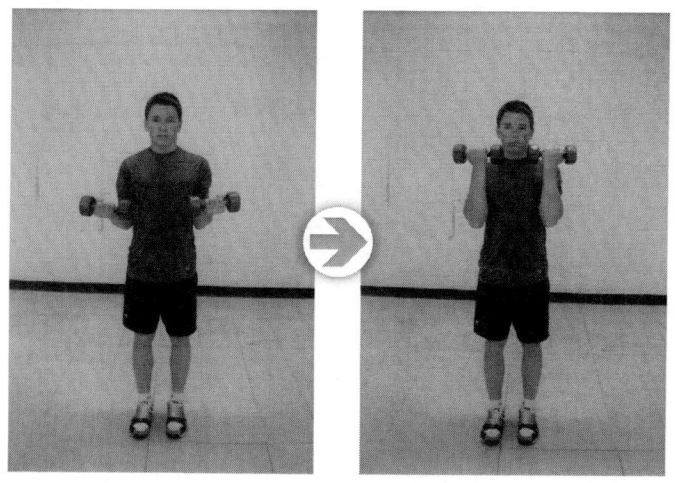

WHAT ARE YOU WAITING FOR?

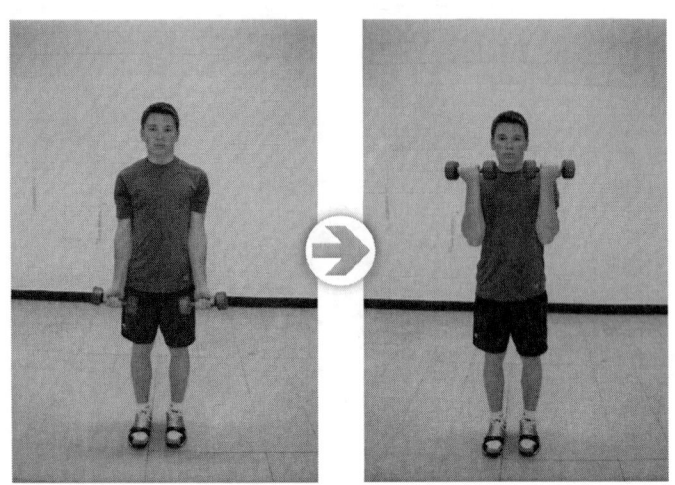

Isolation Curls

Sit on a bench or chair and lean over so that your elbow locks into your thigh, just behind the knee. For this exercise, your arm will hang straight down, and your palm should be aimed towards your opposite leg. Curl the weight up until the head of the dumbbell nearest your pinky touches your chest and then slowly guide it back to the starting position. As with other lifts mentioned, you may find that one side is a little weaker than the other. As before, do your weak side first, so you know how many to do with your strong arm. Over time, it will even out.

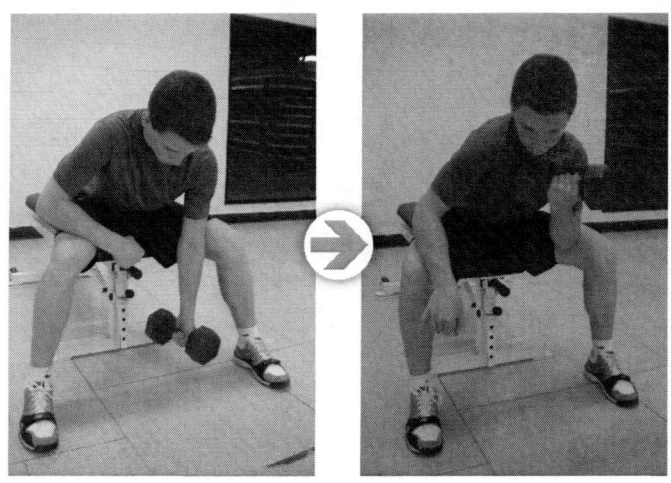

Standing Wall Curls

This is a great exercise to do to get used to the idea of standing and lifting weights. The stance is the same as described before, with the feet shoulder width apart and a slight bend in the knee. With this exercise, you should use a curl bar (as with the preacher curl), but for this exercise, keep your back and elbows against a wall throughout the exercise. Lean slightly into the wall and lift from your waist to your chin then slowly guide the weight back to your waist. This will develop excellent form and not allow you to rock the weight up.

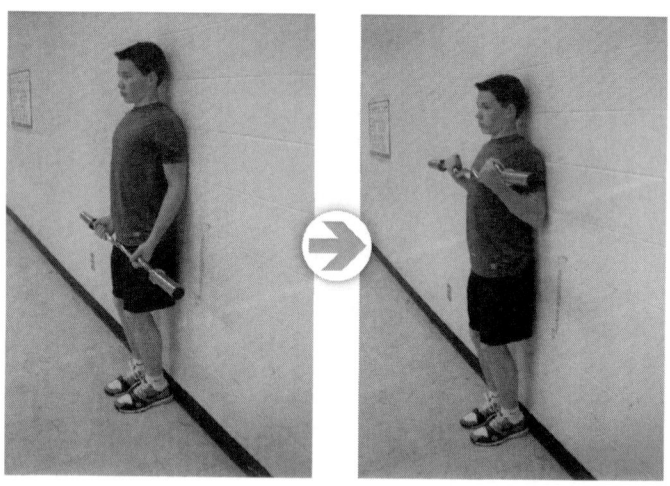

Ten-second Curls

(Set of six at a time)

This is one of my personal favorites. Start on the preacher bench. You will need one of two things here: either a clock with a second hand or a partner to count ten seconds for you. Start with the weight up by your chin and when the second hand reaches twelve or whatever whole number you wish to start at (or your partner says go) *slowly* start to release your arms away from you. When the clock (or your partner) hits the nine-second mark pull it up towards your chin again and immediately start the downward count again. Continue this move for six reps (1 full minute). A word of caution: If you haven't done a lot of weight lifting, you may want to hold off on this one until at least week three of your training. This is a great exercise, but probably a little advanced for just starting out, and it does require some degree of muscular endurance to do this. Once you do begin, you may only be able to get one set. Work your way up to three sets maximum. This is a great exercise to finish a bicep workout.

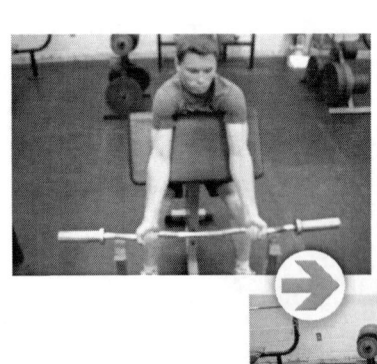

Group Two Stretches

Just like Group One stretches, make sure you have warmed up. As with group one, it is not only important to stretch before but after as well. Go through each of these twice in the warm up and at least twice after completing your workout.

Hamstring Stretch (stretches the hamstring muscles)

Stand with your feet wide apart, knees locked, and toes pointing forward. Lean forward as far as you can without allowing your knees to bend. Your hands can reach for your ankles, between your feet behind you, or just dangle to the floor. Hold for ten to thirty seconds. From this position, try to touch your chest to your left knee and hold for ten to thirty seconds, then do the same stretch to the right and hold.

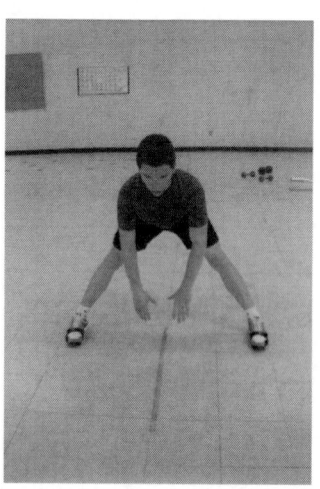

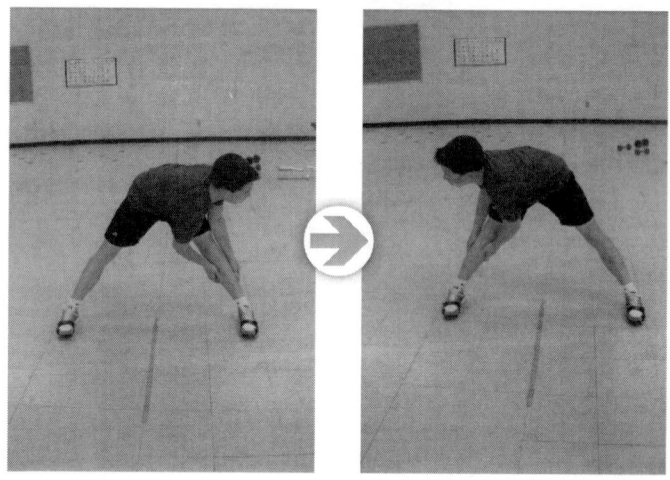

Groin Stretch (stretches the inner thigh muscles)

With your feet wide apart, bend your right leg while keeping your left leg straight and your left foot flat on the ground. Hold for ten to thirty seconds, then slowly move to the left and repeat the move keeping your right leg straight and right foot flat on the ground.

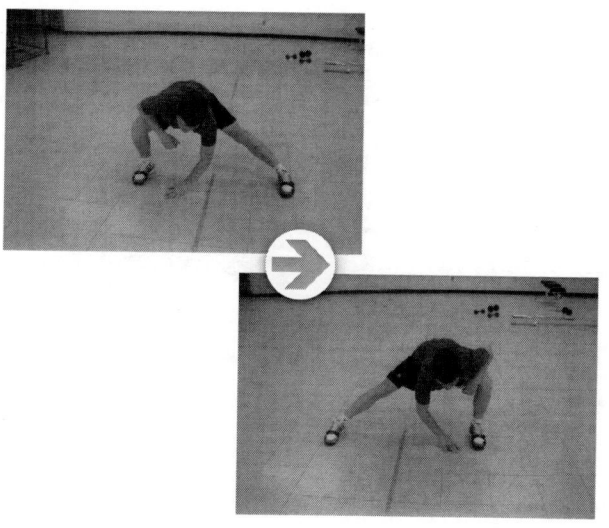

Standing Quad Stretch (stretches the quadriceps muscles)

Stand tall, feet shoulder width apart, grab one leg (you may need help with balance, so use a wall, stool, or whatever) and pull the sole of your shoe up towards your butt. Make sure to stand up tall and keep your bent knee aiming towards the floor (don't let it flare out to the side). Hold for ten to thirty seconds then switch legs.

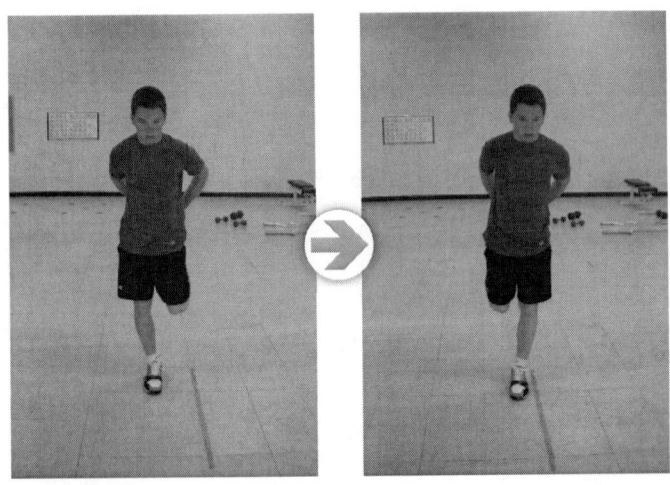

Side Stretch (stretches the lateral muscles)

Stand up tall, both arms raised straight to the sky. Take your right hand and drop it down to your side, lean your left hip out, and lean as far as you can to the right. Keep your left arm straight as you bend, and gently turn your head up so you are looking at your left palm. Hold for ten to thirty seconds and then repeat the move on the other side. You can do this one with your feet close together or shoulder width apart, whichever is more comfortable to you.

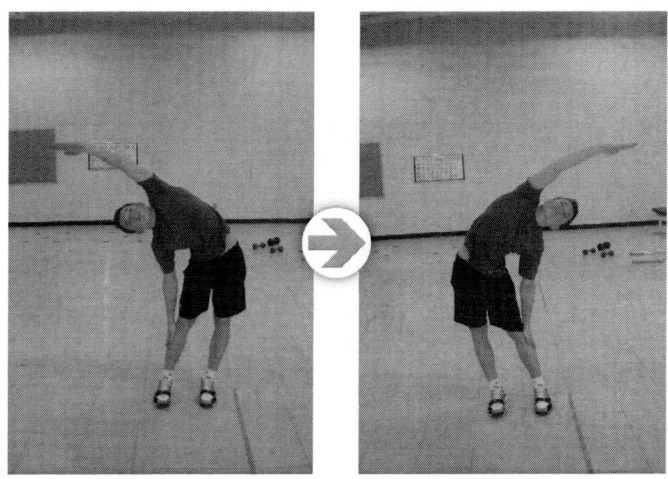

Cobra Stretch (stretches the abdominal muscles)

Lay flat out on your belly, hands up near the shoulders. Press your upper half up into the air, while keeping your hips on the ground. Gently look up, as if you are trying to sneak a peek behind you. If you can't get your arms totally straight before your hips come up too far, then get your arms as straight as possible. Hold for ten to thirty seconds.

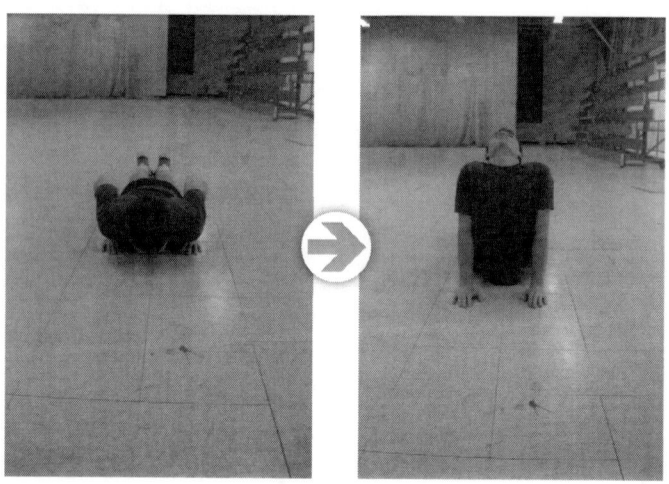

Cat Stretch (stretches the lower back and abdominal muscles)

Start with a flat back on your hands and knees. Your hands should be directly under your shoulders, and your knees directly under your hips. Slowly arch your head up and press your belly towards the floor as you inhale, hold for a moment, then exhale. As you are exhaling, press your back up towards the ceiling. Repeat this two to three times.

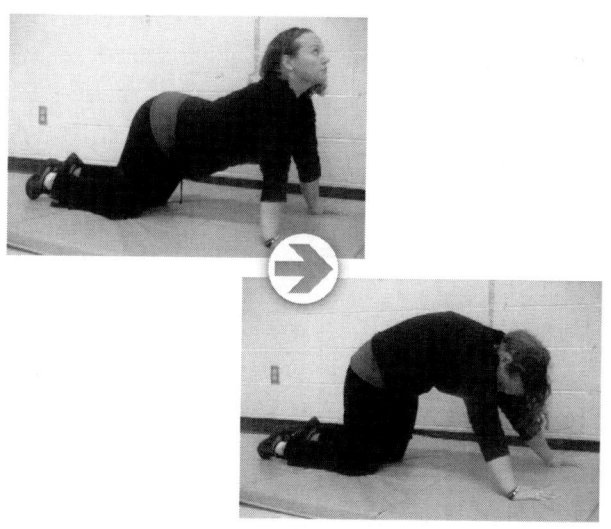

Lats

(Breathing: Exhale the weight towards you, inhale the weight away from you.)

Lawn Mowers

Use a bench that will allow you to keep your foot flat on the floor and your back flat. Placement of the foot that is on the floor isn't critical, but it should be comfortable and help you maintain balance. Allow the bench to hold your body weight. Place your right knee and right hand on the bench. Have the weight in your left hand, arm hanging straight down. As you pull the weight up, allow your elbow to bend so that the head of the weight nearest your thumb is in line with your arm pit. You don't have to actually contact your arm pit with the weight to get a benefit, but raise the weight as close as possible as if it were on a line to that aiming point. Once you have reached the high point of the lift, while keeping your back flat, roll your shoulder blade as if you wanted it to touch your other shoulder. Keep your elbow close to your body as you raise your arm. Slowly guide the weight back to the starting position.

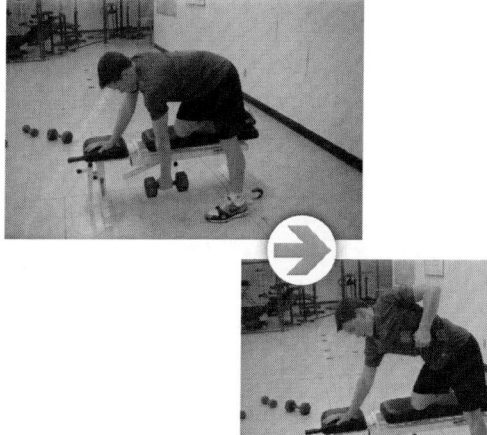

Lat Pull Downs

Before starting this exercise, make sure you have the seat and leg pad adjusted. Set the pad snug enough so that you won't pop out of the seat as the weight is being released, but not so tight that you won't be able to stand back up. You may have to start this exercise standing so that you can get a good grip on the weight. If so, get a good grip on the bar (the wider your hands the better), and slowly guide yourself to the seat and tuck your legs under the pad. Lean back so that you are on an angle somewhere between thirty and forty degrees. Pull the bar to your chest. Slowly guide the weight back to the starting position.

Some words of caution here: when you finish this exercise, do not just release the weight and allow it to slam down. This is bad for equipment and can also lead to injury. To finish, let your arms extend and slowly stand back up as you guide the weight down.

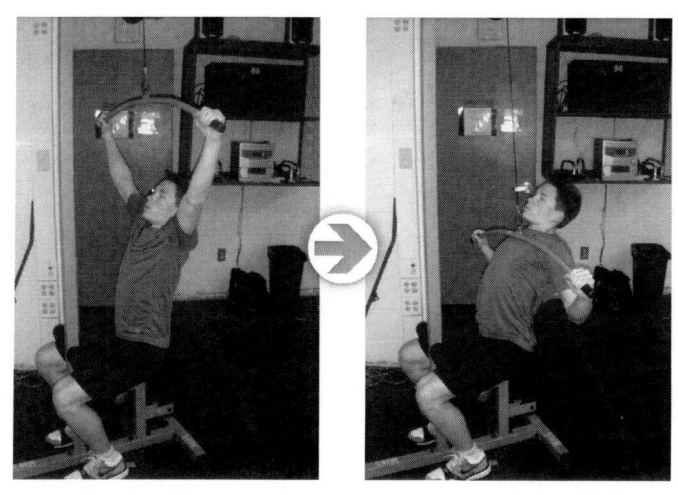

Straight Arm Pull Downs

This exercise is similar to the triceps pull downs, but, as you can see, your elbows don't stay in tight to your body. Keep a slight bend in the elbow to reduce unnecessary strain. Keep your upper body stationary.

You can play with the width of your hands, from shoulder width to a little wider, whatever you feel comfortable with. Once you have set up for this, you may wish to take a step backwards, to keep the weight from hitting during this exercise. It will also allow you a fuller range of motion. The move for this exercise is from eye level to waist, and back to eye level again. Be conscious of keeping just a slight bend in the elbow throughout the whole move. Sometimes, as the bar moves towards the belt line, there is a tendency to bend the elbow in towards the belly button. Make sure that the only joint moving the weight is the shoulder joint, and that your hands extend down to your belt line just below your hips.

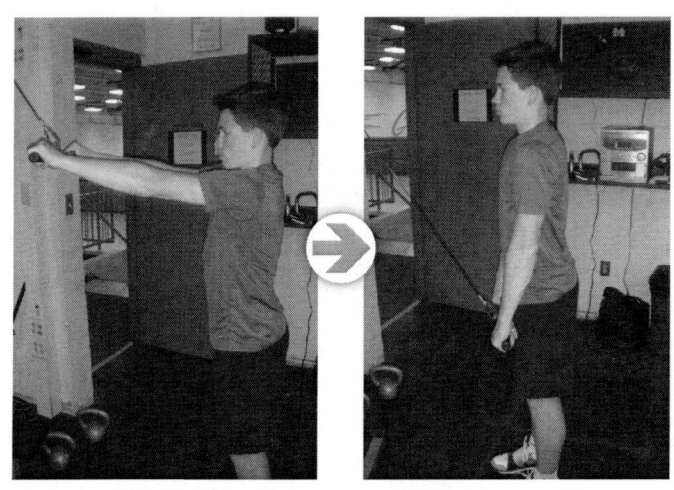

Bent Over Rows

Get a good wide stance for this one (knees slightly bent, of course). This may be difficult at first, as there is a lot to do with balance here, as well. Starting out, use a very lightweight, or even just the bar. With all these lifts, getting the proper technique first is very important. Bend at the waist to as close to ninety degrees as possible. Your grip should be wider than your shoulders, with your palms facing in towards your shins. Bring the bar from straight-arm to the lower portion of your rib cage/upper abdominal area. Slowly guide the weight back down to a straight-arm position. Your elbows should be going back towards your hips, not a "T" like bent over shoulder flies.

If you feel any sort of weirdness in your lower back, stop and check your form (or the amount of weight being used). It is very important to keep your upper body from moving and swaying as you perform this lift, so as to minimize the risk of lower back injury. I can't stress enough the importance of starting light with this lift!

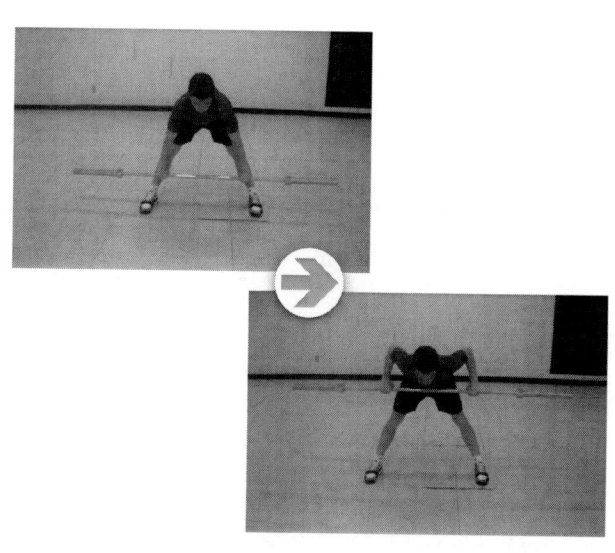

Reverse Grip Bent Over Rows

This is like a bent over row with a slight variation in your hands. For this lift, turn your palms away from your legs. Everything else is the same as the regular bent over row, except that your aiming point should be your belly button. This is a great lift for really blasting the lower third of your Lateralis muscles.

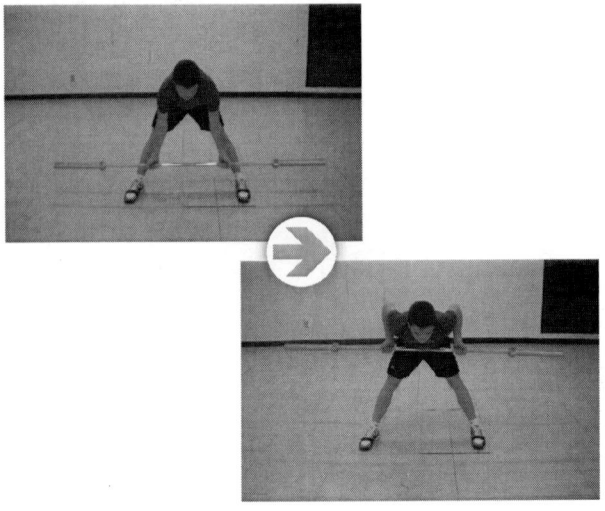

Seated Rows

This is very much like a bent over row, except, of course, now you are on your butt. Use the "V" bar instead of the long straight bar used for pull downs (notice the hand placement on the bar…this avoids wrist strain). As you can also see, you want to pull both hands back to your belly button. This will give you enough bend in the elbows to get deep into the Lateralis muscles.

You should also (as you see) lean forward as you bring your arms straight, and lean back as you pull the weight towards you to increase the range of motion with this exercise. As you pull, keep the elbows close to your sides to help isolate the lats.

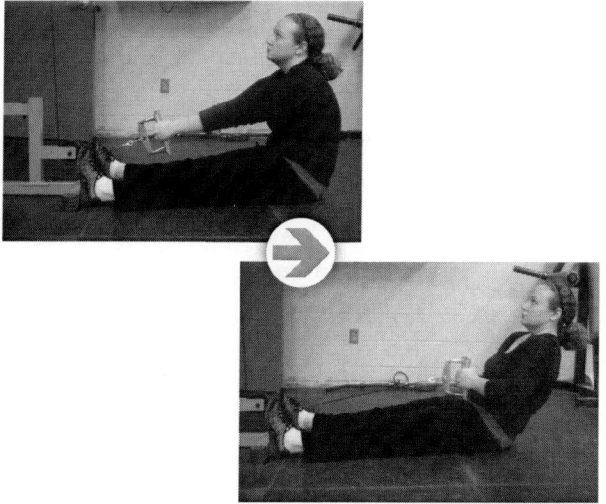

Quads

(Breathing: Exhale the weight up, inhale as you bring it down.)

Leg Extension

Proper placement of the leg pad is key. Set it up so that the pad rests in the nook between your ankle and shin. Make sure to keep your back straight (whether your machine has a back rest or not), and also use the handlebars (99 percent of all extension machines have them) to help keep your butt on the seat. If the backrest is adjustable, set it up so that the edge of the chair is touching behind your knees. If you cannot adjust the backrest, then sit so that your knees are bending right at the edge of the seat. This is also a key point to proper form. Everything from your knee down should be below the seat.

Starting with your legs in the down position, kick the weight forward until your shins are parallel with the ground. Now, at this point, many people (wrongly) slam the weight back down. That's a bad idea. Not only can you break the machine, but you really don't get the work done doing this. Slowly guide the weight back to the starting position.

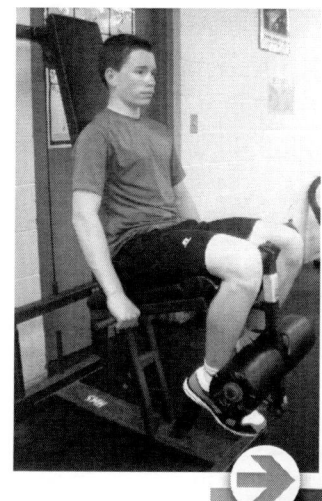

Wall Sits

(Minimum one minute each.)

If legwork is new to you, this one may take a little time to develop, but it is a great way to build leg strength quickly. There are many variations of this to help you develop this skill.

The goal for this exercise is to sit for one minute, back tight against the wall, knees bent to ninety degrees, knees lined up directly over your ankles, arms straight out in front of you, or palms flat against the wall. It's your choice. Now, that sounds easy enough, but I guarantee you it is a lot harder than it sounds. As far as sets for this exercise, work your way up to three to four one minute sets. In the beginning, you may only get thirty seconds or less and need a break. Go ahead take it! Take a second or two and shake out your legs, then get right back to it. Some things you could do if you find the full one minute difficult would be to do twenty seconds on, ten off, twenty on, ten off. Then move to thirty second on, ten off. Over time, work your way up to the full minute. Another idea would be that you could go to the ninety degree point for twenty seconds, then raise up to a (roughly) forty-five degree angle for ten seconds, and then back down to ninety degrees for twenty. Whatever gets you started. Remember, the goal is to eventually hold it for one minute.

Once you have mastered three to four one minute sets you can challenge yourself by placing a weight in your lap or against your chest for more challenge. You could also do one-legged wall sits, where you keep one leg bent at ninety degrees, and try to hold the other one straight out and parallel to the floor switching legs every ten seconds. There is a lot you can do with this one, so once you have it down use your imagination to challenge yourself.

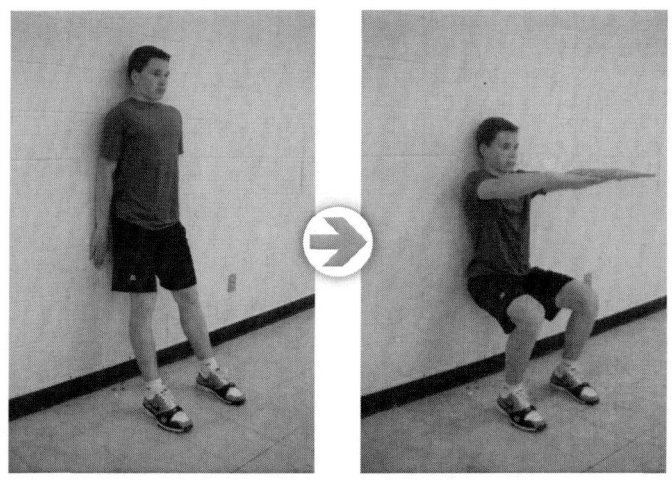

Dumbbell Squat

The form described here will be very much like the squat, which you will hear about a little later. Until you have things a little bit figured out, start with a very light weight. This is a great way to get the form down for proper barbell squats.

Start with your feet in the usual shoulder width apart. Slightly angle your toes out for balance. Keep a slight bend in the knee. Make sure your back stays straight all throughout this exercise (no bending at the hip!). To help with this, it is a good idea to pick a spot on the wall just above your head (so you are staring up at a roughly forty-five-degree angle). Keep your eyes on this spot the whole time. Hold the weights firmly in your hands, but keep your arms straight. Bend at the knees until you have a roughly ninety-degree angle, and then return to the starting position. You may be able to, but there is no good that can come from bending farther than ninety degrees.

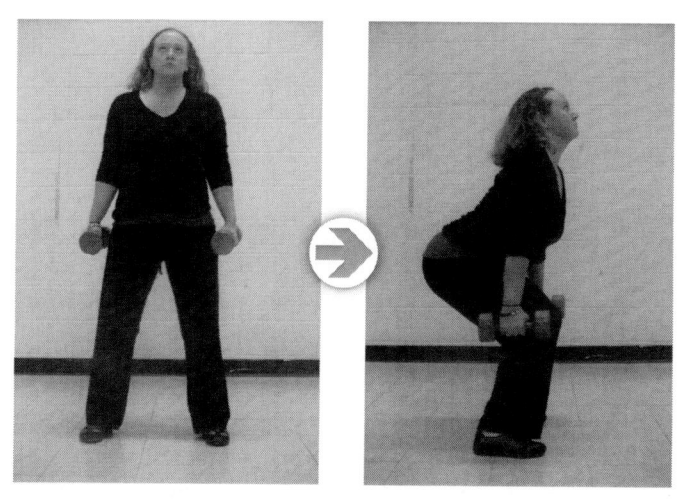

Hamstring

(Breathing: Exhale the weight up, inhale as you bring it down.)

Leg Curls

As with leg extensions, pad placement is key to doing this exercise correctly. Make sure that the pads are on your Achilles tendon, just above your heel. Having them elsewhere will result in not getting a full range of motion.

Starting with your legs straight, pull the weight up to your butt. As you pull the weight up, concentrate on keeping your belly on the table and your head in the neutral position (no arch or bow in the back). Then, slowly guide it back down. Also, if they are available, using the handles will help keep you from arching.

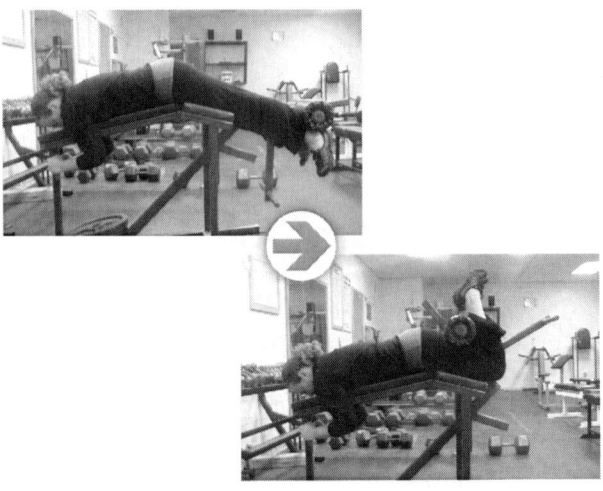

Straight Leg Dead Lift

Start with your stance a bit wider than shoulder width apart. Even though the name is Straight Leg, do not fully lock your knees out. To start, if possible, have the weight set up so that you can pick it up at about waist level. If not, you can pick it up from the floor, but make sure to lift it properly with your legs, keeping your back straight. It is also worth mentioning (as you can imagine) that until you have this down, start with a very light weight to work the proper form.

Allow the weight to dangle in your hands, but maintain a good, solid grip. Bend slowly forward at the waist until you reach the ninety-degree mark and then slowly stand back up. You may have to play with your leg width to maintain balance. The object here is to get to ninety degrees, not to have the weights hit the floor with every rep. If, at any point, you feel a tweak in your lower back, put the weight up and start with a lighter set.

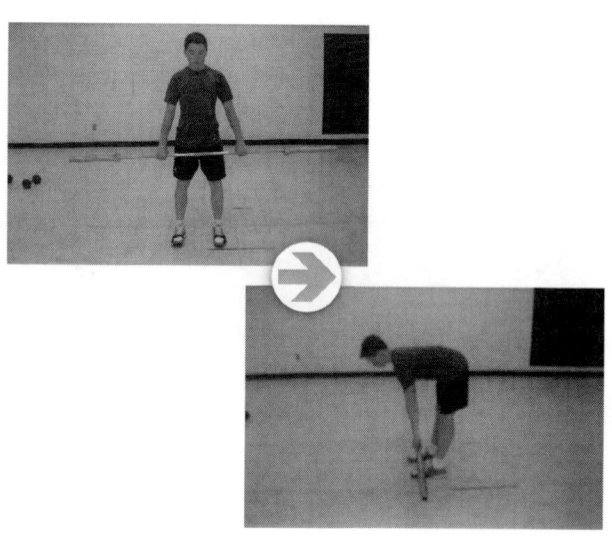

Good Mornings

The only difference between good mornings and the straight leg dead lift is the placement of the weight. Both are excellent for isolating the hamstring muscles. One thing you might find different is that, with the weight higher for good mornings, your balance will need some work. Lastly, you will probably need to start with a lighter weight than with straight leg dead lifts due to the change in your center of gravity.

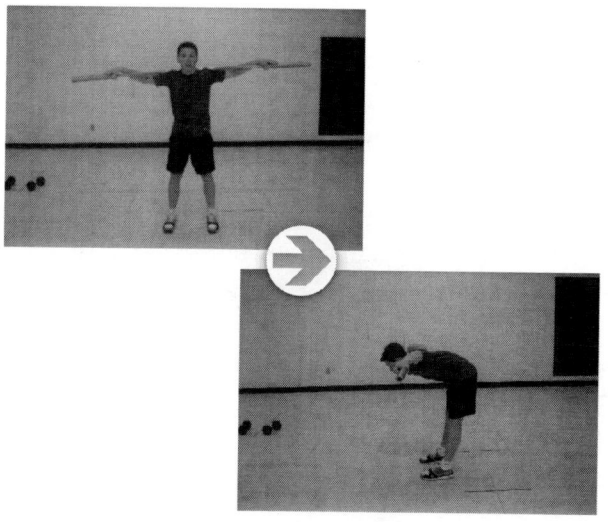

Flutter Kicks

(Up to one minute per set.)

Lay out flat on the floor (or mat if you want a little more comfort). Basically, this is just like a free-style swimming kick. Keep your legs straight, and get as much of your legs off the ground as possible while you work (nothing but hips on the floor is best). It is very important to keep your head in the neutral position to avoid a neck strain. As for your arms, you could either place them by your side, or put them out in front of you, whichever you find more comfortable.

This is an exercise similar to Wall Sits, in that you can play with the time as far as set length. Keep your set maximum to four, and work towards one-minute sets. To start, work for however many sets it takes for you to get two full minutes of work done, meaning that if you stop to take a break, stop the time during your minute sets. Build up from there. Make sure that as you kick you are moving from the hips, not the knees. If you feel this move in your lower back, gluteus muscles, and hamstrings, you are doing it right.

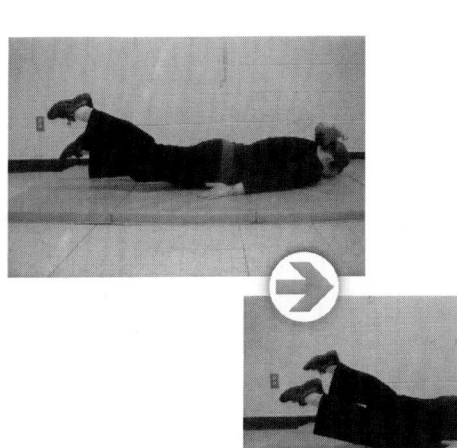

Leg Combo

Squats

Having read the form for dumbbell squats, you know the proper stance. One difference is that now you will have the weight on your back. Make sure that the barbell is at the base of your neck, and resting on top of your shoulders. Balance could be an issue, so, as mentioned before, start light to get the form down.

As with the bench press, having a spotter is necessary for this. No matter what, this exercise should not be done if you don't have a spotter.

To review, your legs should be shoulder width apart, toes very slightly angled out, and knees slightly bent. Bend at the knees until you reach the ninety-degree mark and return to the starting position. Remember to pick a spot on the wall to keep your eyes on to help keep your back straight.

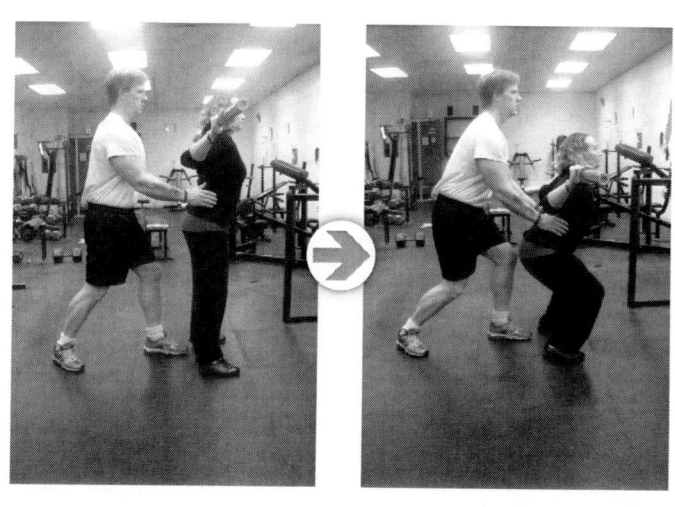

Plyometric Jumps

(One set = one minute.)

This exercise is similar to wall sits and flutter kicks, in that you can control the amount you do during the time limit. For this exercise, keep the time at one minute per set. As you progress with your workouts, you can work on increasing the intensity by increasing the height of each individual jump and amount of jumps you do per set.

Each jump should be its own separate movement. What I mean by this is that you should come to a *complete* stop and wind up in the start/finish position before jumping again.

The start/finish position is a ninety-degree bend in the knees, head up, back straight, and arms back in the launch position. When you jump, swing your arms up and reach as high above your head as possible. Land as quietly as possible on the balls of your feet. As your feet land, recoil your body back to the start/finish position. Make sure you are completely stopped and reset before jumping again.

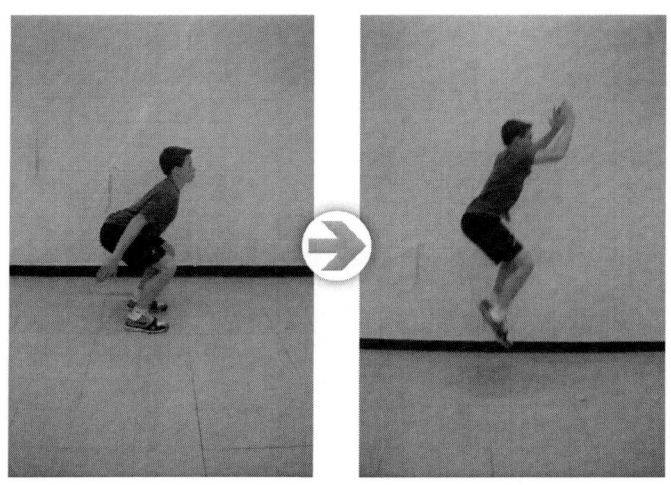

Lunges

Initially, you may find that doing this move without any weight is plenty. The big key to this is slow, quality movement. Speeding through this exercise won't really help you get better. To start, stand with your feet together; back straight, head up looking straight ahead of you. If you choose to use weight, keep your arms straight and let the weight dangle.

Step straight out in front of you with your left leg. Make sure to keep your right leg planted (although you will naturally lift your heel, which is fine, but don't allow the toes to move from their place) and make sure the right leg stays straight. As for how far to step out, you should take a little larger than normal stride (somewhere between thirty to thirty-six inches). From here, bend the left knee until you reach the ninety-degree mark. At this point, you have two options. You could do walking lunges, which means that as you straighten your left leg, you bring your right leg up to it, moving forward as you do. You could also do stationary lunges, in which when you begin to straighten your left leg, you push up hard, and bring your left foot back next to your right foot. Repeat this move on the other side. As you step out, whether walking or stationary style, maintain the straight back, eyes forward form throughout. One last thing here: a set of ten means ten on each leg, not ten total!

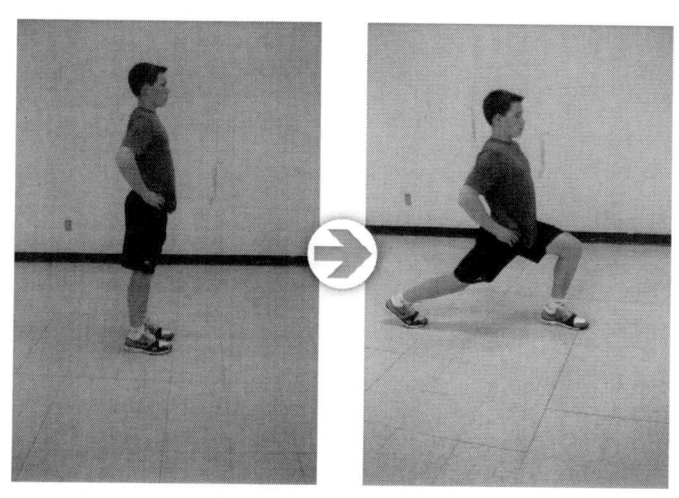

Side Lunges

For this style of lunge, stand with your feet together, head up, back straight, and eyes forward. Keeping your body facing forward, step sideways (about 30-36 inches) with your left leg, keeping your right leg straight (you will naturally roll onto the inside of your foot). Once your left knee gets to the ninety-degree mark, explode yourself upwards and bring your left foot back to your right one. Repeat this move on the right side.

If you are using weights for this one, as you move to the left the weight in your right hand should move and be lowered between your feet. The weight in your left hand should stay to the outside. Reverse this when you move to the right. Counting reps is the same as the lunges previously described.

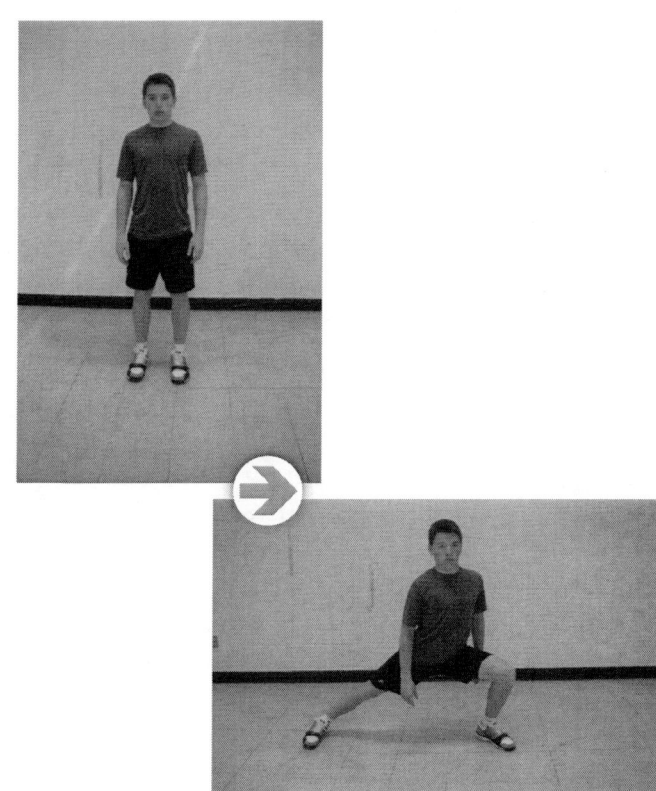

Abdominals

(Breathing: exhale up, inhale down.)

None of these will or should fit the two to four sets of ten or 12-15 routine. To start, pick as many exercises as you want to do for the day (at least three separate moves, but more would be ok also), and do as many sets necessary to complete 150 abdominal moves. As an example, 50 Russian twists, 50 bicycle twists, 50 feet up crunch. Something like that. As you work remember to mix it up, meaning don't continually do the same few exercises. We all have favorite moves, but variety here is a good thing not only for abs, but for all muscle groups.

Over time, you will find that you can do more per set to get to the 150 mark. Eventually, work your rep number up from 150 to 300-350. Take as many sets as you need to in order to accomplish this. Start slow and work your way up. As you gain more confidence and experience, shorten your rest period from the usual one to two minutes to fifteen seconds to no longer than one minute.

Russian Twists

As shown, these are being done off the ground. If you want to, as you get more comfortable with this move, you could use a flat bench, so that you can get your legs over even farther. To begin, lay flat on your back with your hands above your head, and (as shown) hold onto something permanent to give you a solid base.

Start with your feet up in the air, legs as straight as possible (photo 1). As you roll to one side, get directly onto your hip, and move your legs from the ninety-degree starting position to about thirty degrees as you guide your feet towards the floor (photo 2). Don't allow your feet to actually touch the floor (stop somewhere between one and four inches above the ground). From here, bring your feet back to the starting position and roll to the other side (photo 3). Once you get started with this exercise, you won't stop at the top of the move, but rather you should lift your butt into the sky, to help you in rolling onto your other hip (photo 4). Make sure that only your lower half, from hips to feet, are moving throughout this move. Keep your shoulders flat on the floor as you roll to isolate the abs. As with the lunges, a set of ten consists of ten on each side.

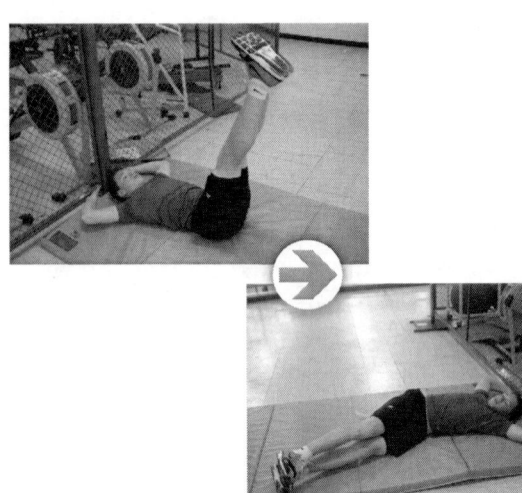
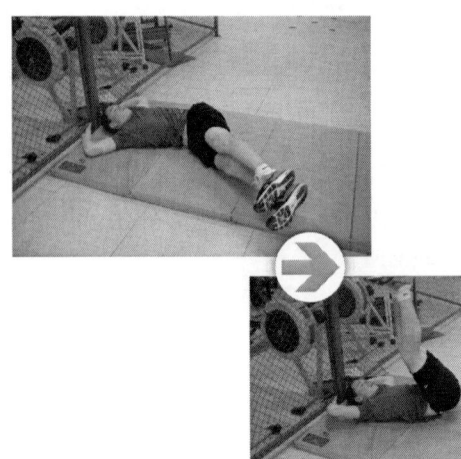

Feet Up Crunch

This is the traditional crunch that most people think of, but I want to explain the proper way of doing this. By raising your legs, you will be focusing more intensity on the abdominal area. Doing a bent knee sit-up or crunch with your feet on the floor will work your hip-pointer more than your abs. I prefer (as the picture shows) to use the cross arm method. Many people who clasp their hands behind their head (whether knowingly or unknowingly) pull themselves up and not only cheat , but risk neck strain by pulling so hard. Another option with your hands would be to lay them palms down by your side, and slide them forward on the floor as you lift your shoulders up.

To properly do a crunch, all that needs to come up off the floor are your shoulder blades. Once you get the upper part of your back off the ground, hold for about one second, and then slowly lower yourself back to the floor. One thing you will find is that the closer your knees are to ninety degrees, the tougher the move will be.

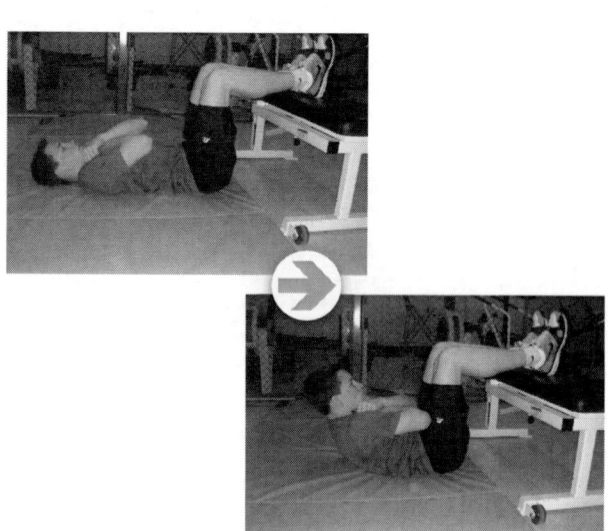

Leg Lifts

Lie flat on the ground, legs straight. I prefer to put my hands under my hips to help reduce lower back strain. Start with your feet about an inch off the ground. Keeping your butt on the floor, raise your legs to ninety degrees, and slowly lower them to about one inch off the ground.

As you begin this exercise, you may find that you have a tendency to want to bend your knees as you bring your legs up. Be conscious that, as you raise your legs, your knees stay locked to keep your legs straight. Also, keep your head flat on the ground in the neutral position throughout the movement. You could point your toes or keep your feet flat, whatever feels more comfortable to you.

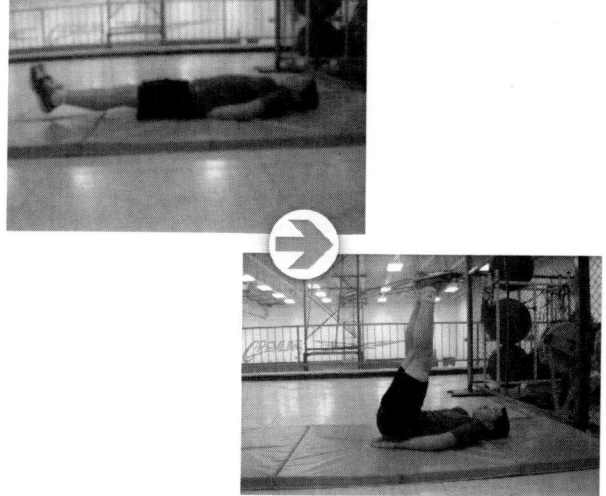

Bicycle Twist Crunch

Lie flat out on your back. You can either use the cross-arm method or, if it feels a little more comfortable, place your hands on the side of your head over your ears (*not* clasped together behind your head or neck!). Get your feet about an inch or so off the floor, and, one leg at a time, bend your knee up as close to your chest as possible. At the same time, twist your body to try and touch your opposite elbow to your bent knee (right elbow to left knee, left elbow to right knee).

The upper half of your body will more or less roll from one side to the other (make sure to get the shoulder blades off the ground as you reach and twist). Your legs should come straight up towards your chest as high as you can reach them. If your elbow touches your knee that's great flexibility and abdominal strength, but it is not necessary to have them touch to see a benefit. Making the effort with each repetition is the important thing. One twist to each side equals one rep.

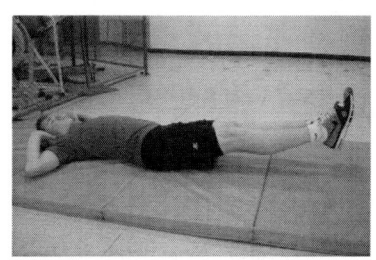

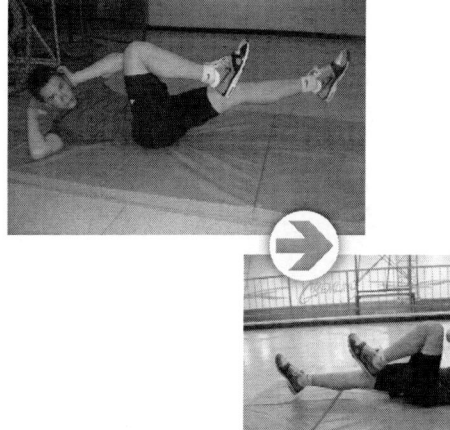

Heel Lifts

For this exercise, you may place your hands in one of three spots. Either at your side, palms down under your hips, or above your head holding something (like Russian twists) to help steady you. The movement you want for this exercise is to lift your lower end up far enough off the floor to get your hips totally off the ground.

As you move, be conscious to not point your toes. Keep your knees locked and legs straight. Your heels should go *straight* up in the air, not up towards your head or upper body. To help with this upward movement, squeeze your butt together. This will also help to keep your movement straight.

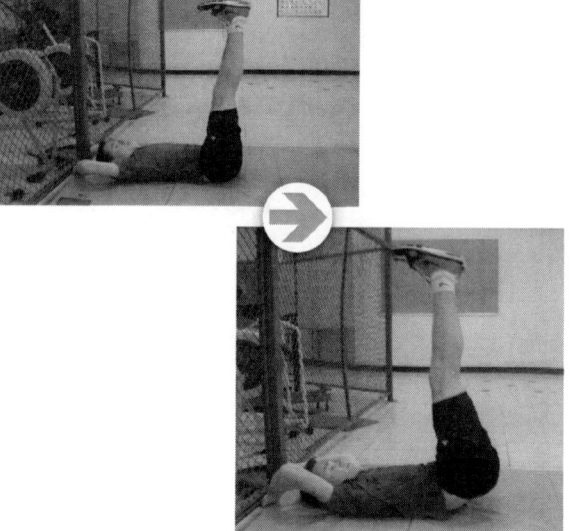

Side Crunch

Lay on your side, legs at about a thirty-degree angle to your torso. Place your upper hand on the back of your head, lower hand palm down on the ground, against your body. Try to touch your elbow to your thigh by raising both your legs and shoulder up. Making contact with your thigh and elbow is great, but not necessary (as with bicycle twists). Make an honest effort and over time you will improve. Remember how many you do, because you will have to do that many on the other side. As for counting, this exercise is like lunges. Let's say you do twenty-five on each side, you should only count twenty-five towards your total count of abdominal work, not fifty.

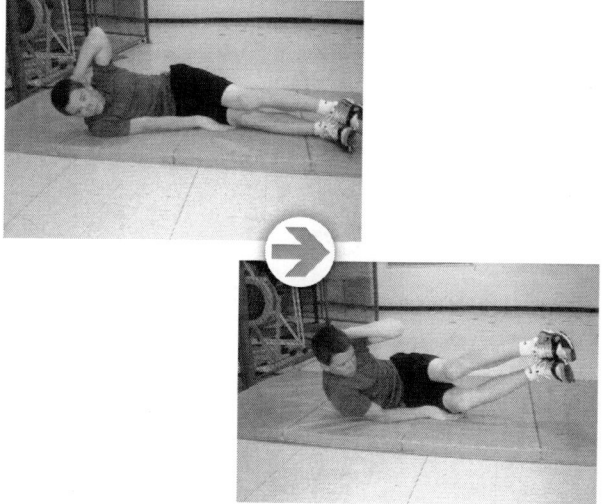

Leg Climb

To start, bend one knee (the closer your foot is to your butt the tougher each rep will be). With your other leg, place it up in the air in about a forty-five-degree angle. Take as many grabs as necessary to climb to your foot, and then slowly lower back to the ground. The less grabs the harder it will be. Keep track of how many you do per side. If you do 10 on each leg, then that's 10 towards the total.

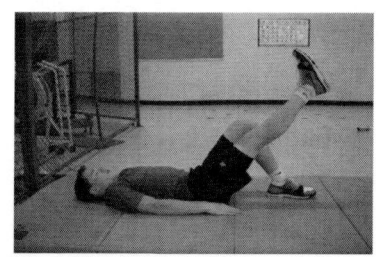

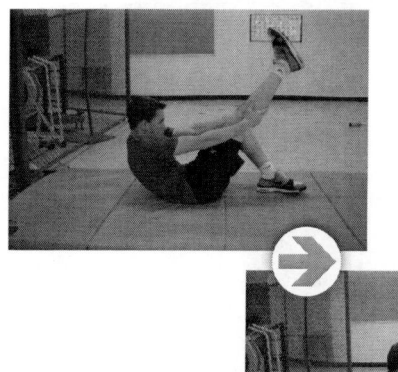

VARIATION

As I mentioned earlier, along with weight training, you should also do some sort of cardiovascular exercise. I thought I would throw this next section in to combine both weight lifting and cardio. This training is a form of circuit training. One disadvantage of this is that, since there really is no rest period, you need to have a nearly empty weight room. Efficiency of movement is a key to keep the heart rate up. One big advantage of this is kind of the same reason. Since there is no rest period, you can get a good cardio workout in as you lift.

Before you set off on a circuit, make sure you have all your weights set and ready to reduce the amount of time between sets. You will find that by working a circuit, your time in the gym is shorter, but you can still get a great work out. Something else to consider here is that you don't want to do something like this on a full stomach. Continual work like this can lead to cramps or even worse, and getting sick is not worth whatever you ate. I would recommend a water bottle though (as with any workout, keeping hydrated is very important).

To start, pick three different exercises from each category in each group. Perform your lifts in this order (I will start with Group One) *Chest, Biceps, Triceps, Shoulders*. Your goal is to go through each muscle group four times (by picking only three exercises, you will do the first four twice). As you do each exercise, make sure that you are using the proper techniques for each movement. There is no reason to rush through each lift. The speed for this type of exercise program comes from the no rest period between sets, not from racing through each individual lift as fast as possible. This is more of a toning/muscle building/fat burning workout, so keep each set somewhere between twelve and fifteen. For Group One, you will perform sixteen total exercises.

After you get your weights set up, go through the proper warm up and stretch for the group you are going to work. Once you are ready, get started, and don't stop until you have all your lifts done. I *highly* recommend that for this type of workout you write down exactly what exercises you want to do before you get started. I have tried to do this from memory and usually it gets screwed up. Take my advice on this one and save yourself the frustration and trouble and write it down. Here is a sample of a Circuit workout:

1. Bench Press
2. Preacher Curls
3. Dips
4. Lateral Raises
5. Pec Deck Fly Machine
6. One-Arm Standing Full Supination Curls
7. Triceps Pull Downs
8. Military Press
9. Incline Bench Press
10. Hammer Curls
11. Throw Backs
12. Wide Grip Upright Rows
13. Bench Press
14. Preacher Curls
15. Dips
16. Lateral Raise

A Group Two circuit would be a little different, in that throughout the workout, you would do the same two quad and hamstring exercises, but vary the rest. The order would be like this: *Quads, Hamstrings, Lats, Leg Combo, and Abdominals*. Work each muscle group four times. As for abs, you could go about it a few different ways. You could do a set number each time abs come up (say, twenty-five), you could go for a certain length of time per abdominal exercise (maybe thirty to sixty seconds), or when it comes time for the abdominals section, you could go to failure. If you have a thought, go for it! Experiment and see what you like the best and what is best for you. An example list would look like this:

1. Leg Extension
2. Leg Curls
3. Lawn Mowers
4. Lunges
5. Bent Knee Crunch
6. Leg Extension
7. Leg Curls
8. Lat Pull Downs
9. Plyometric Jumps
10. Bicycle Twist Crunch
11. Leg Extension
12. Leg Curls
13. Bent Over Rows
14. Squats
15. Leg Lifts
16. Leg Extension

17. Leg Curls
18. Lawn Mowers
19. Lunges
20. Bent Knee Crunch

You may find that by doing a workout like this, at least initially, you can't quite get through all the lifts without stopping. I remember the first circuit workout I ever did. It took me about two weeks to get through a workout without feeling like I was going to throw up and another two weeks to get through the workout without stopping.

If you have to stop, keep your breaks short (no more than thirty to sixty seconds). Take them at the end (if possible) of each cycle. A cycle would be after each major muscle group has been accomplished (for Group One, the cycles end with four, eight, twelve, and sixteen, Group Two—five, ten, fifteen, and twenty). Work towards no breaks through the whole workout.

AND FINALLY...

So, there you have it. Not only do you now have a great grasp of the basics of lifting but you even have a whole separate workout to challenge you! As mentioned throughout this book, this is a beginning for you. This will give you the basics. This will get you started. This should not be seen as the "be all, end all" of weight training (although, if you choose to, everything in here will fit you for the rest of your life and help you to reach your goals). This should be the kicker that gets you off the couch and no longer will allow you to use the excuse, "I would love to get started, but I don't know where to begin."

As time goes by and you begin to gain more confidence, you should add to your routine and learn some other lifts. I like to change my routine up every so often so that it doesn't get old and boring. Remember, though, learn the proper techniques first. I continue to try new and different things to keep challenging myself. This should be seen as your starting point. After a few weeks when you feel you are getting the hang of things, something basic to change up your routine a little would be to start with a different muscle group first. It seems simple, but we all develop habits when we workout, and sometimes just starting at a different point is enough of a challenge.

I want to thank you for investing your time and money into purchasing this book. Where you go from here is totally up to you. I hope that you use this information to change your life. I would hate to think that you spent this much time learning and then just stopped without ever really giving yourself a chance. One final bit of knowledge I want to pass on to you is something I learned from a coach of mine long ago (it is more a philosophy of life that I have tried to live by). "When it comes to getting better and improving in anything, whether it is sports, education, relationships, or what have you, it will take four things from the person who wishes to change: effort, courage, discipline, and enthusiasm." Put these four words into your life and your exercise routine and you will see major change.

I think it's worth mentioning one final time here that the only thing holding you back is *your* work ethic and *your* motivation to change! I know, I said that earlier, but I want to stress that point. It is totally up to you what you do now with the knowledge you have gained. I wish you well!

APPENDIX

As I was writing this book, I noticed that I mentioned the importance of writing down and tracking your workouts several times. It occurred to me how easy it would be to include this part for you, so that you can photo copy this sheet as much as necessary to start your workout journal. I also recommend writing down anything you think valuable in the comments: how you felt, whether a weight was too heavy or too light, or anything you want to keep track of. Not only will this help you in reaching your goals, but it will also allow you to see how far you have come as time goes on.

Group One Lifts

Day of Week:

Chest:

Exercise	Weight Used	Reps

Shoulders:

Exercise	Weight Used	Reps

Triceps:

Exercise	Weight Used	Reps

Biceps:

Exercise	Weight Used	Reps

Comments:

Group Two Lifts

Day of Week:

Lats:

Exercise   Weight Used   Reps

_____
_____
_____

Quads:

Exercise   Weight Used   Reps

_____
_____
_____

Hamstrings:

Exercise   Weight Used   Reps

_____
_____
_____
_____

Leg Combo:

Exercise	Weight Used	Reps

Abdominals:

Exercise	Weight Used	Reps

Comments: